CARDIOLOGY HANDBOOK FOR HEALTH PROFESSIONALS

M. Wayne Cooper, M.D.

Section of Cardiology
Texas Tech University
School of Medicine

WARREN H. GREEN, INC.
St. Louis, Missouri, U.S.A.

Published by

WARREN H. GREEN, INC.
8356 Olive Boulevard
St. Louis, Missouri 63132, U.S.A.

ISBN No. 87527-366-1

ACKNOWLEDGMENTS

The author wishes to acknowledge the expert technical help of several individuals during the preparation of this manuscript including Ms. Ann Tapp, Ms. Nancy Frances, Ms. Pam Reed, Ms. Mary Helen Beck, Mr. Victor Maldonado, and, for her help in reviewing and typing this manuscript, Ms. Jo Ethridge.

CONTENTS

CARDIOLOGY HANDBOOK FOR HEALTH PROFESSIONALS

Chapter 1

ANATOMY AND PHYSIOLOGY OF THE CARDIOVASCULAR SYSTEM

FUNCTION

The heart has the task of providing oxygenated blood to all of the vital organs of the body. It must do this continuously, 24 hours a day, for a lifetime. So it serves as a *pump* providing substrate and oxygen, for the body's metabolic processes. If the heart pump weakens, virtually all of the other vital organs are affected. The kidney, which maintains body homeostasis, may respond by retaining more salt and water in order to maintain perfusion pressure. The brain's function may be impaired, resulting in confusion and disorientation. Other vital structures may become engorged with blood, impairing their ability to function.

The heart is an extremely *durable* organ. It normally beats 70 times a minute, 4,200 times an hour, 100,800 times a day, 36,792,000 times a year, or 2,575,409,000 times an average 70–year lifetime. Under conditions of maximal exercise, the heart rate of a young adult may accelerate to 200 beats/minute for several minutes; or, during sleep, this same pump may slow to 40 beats/minute and still maintain adequate output. This same healthy young adult's heart normally pumps 5 liters (1.25 gal) of blood per minute. By the same mathematics, this equals 651,000 gallons/year or 45,900,000 gallons in a lifetime. It takes over three days for an equivalent volume of water to pass over Niagara Falls.

The heart is *unique* in having its own inherent *automaticity*, i.e., the ability to generate an electrical impulse which stimulates the contraction of the pump. These automatic cells may be modulated by external signals but will continue to generate a driving impulse even in the denervated transplanted heart. This system provides a significant safety factor and keeps the heart pumping even if other vital functions are impaired.

ANATOMY OF THE HEART

The heart is a cone-shaped hollow, muscular organ weighing about 300 grams in the adult or about the same size as a closed fist. It is located in the *mediastinum*, a space between the lungs within the thoracic cavity. The base of the cone is directed toward the body's right side. Its apex is directed toward the left and rests upon the diaphragm.

The heart is a double pump having two sides. The *right* side receives deoxygenated blood from the body and pumps it to the lungs to be oxygenated; the *left* side receives oxygenated blood from the lungs and pumps it out through the aorta to all parts of the body (Figure 1.1).

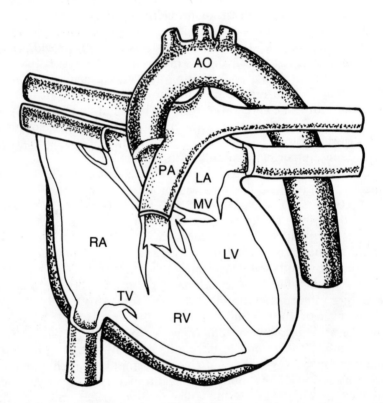

Figure 1.1. Abbreviations: RA = right atrium; TV = tricuspid valve; RV = right ventricle; PA = pulmonary artery, AO = aorta; LA = left atrium; MV = mitral valve; LV = left ventricle.

The heart is enclosed in a sac, the pericardium, a loose fitting covering composed of:

1. *Fibrous pericardium*, a tough fibrous membrane which is attached over the top of the heart to the great vessels.
2. *Serous pericardium* which lines the inside of the fibrous sac and covers the outside of the heart. It is composed of two layers, a) an outer parietal layer that lines the fibrous pericardium and b) an inner visceral layer, the *epicardium* that adheres closely to the heart.

In a healthy state, the two serous membranes are closely opposed to each other, separated only by enough serous or watery fluid to make their surfaces slippery. This lubricates the heart's surfaces and alleviates friction between the surfaces as the heart beats. Since the two surfaces are not attached, there is a potential space between them called the *pericardial cavity.*

After injury or disease, fluid may exude into the cavity causing a wide separation between the heart and the pericardium, producing a *pericardial effusion.*

Component Parts of the Heart

The heart consists of four systems: 1) the pump, 2) the valves, 3) the fuel delivery system (coronary vessels), and 4) the electrical system (conduction system).

The Pump

The Layers of the Cardiac Muscle are:

1. *Epicardium* - outer layer, same structure as visceral pericardium.
2. *Myocardium* - middle layer, composed of striated muscle fibers, interlaced together into bundles. This muscle causes the heart's contraction, which squeezes blood out of the heart into the atrial system.
3. *Endocardium* - innermost layer, composed of endothelial tissue and continuous with the blood vessels. It lines the heart's cavities and covers the heart valves.

The Cardiac Chambers are:

1. *Atria* - the two upper "receiving" chambers. The *right atrium* receives deoxygenated blood from all over the body via the superior and inferior venae cavae, and pumps blood into the right ventricle. From here it is pumped to the lungs for oxygenation.

The *left atrium* receives the oxygenated blood via pulmonary veins from the lungs and pumps it into the left ventricle from which it is pumped out to the body. The two atria are separated by the interarterial septum.

2. *Ventricles* - the two lower "distributing" chambers. The inner wall of the ventricles is characterized by: *trabeculae carnae* - interlacing bundles of muscle; *papillary muscles* - finger or nipple-shaped projections; and *chordae tendinae* - chordlike structures (composed of dense fibrous connective tissue) that are attached to the valve leaflets.

The *right ventricle* receives blood from the right atrium, and pumps it out to the lungs via the *pulmonary artery.*

The *left ventricle* (the heart's largest, most muscular chamber) receives oxygenated blood from the lungs via the left atrium, and pumps it out to all parts of the body.

The *interventricular septum* separates the two ventricles and normally performs as part of the left ventricle.

The Valves

There are a total of four cardiac valves (Figure 1.2).

The Atrioventricular Valves i.e., the tricuspid and bicuspid (mitral) are the valves which guard openings between the atria and ventricles, forcing blood to flow forward from atria to ventricles,

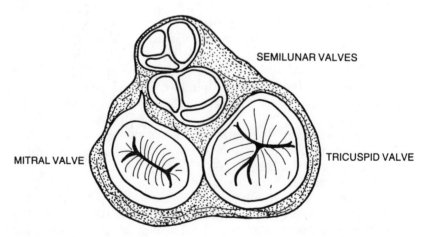

Figure 1.2.

and preventing blood from flowing backward from ventricles to atria. The *tricuspid valve* guards the opening between the right atrium and right ventricle. This is composed of three cusps (flaps) of endothelium. When the right ventricle begins to contract, the pressure rise forces the cusps to close and unite to prevent backward flow of blood. The *bicuspid (mitral) valve* guards the opening between the left atrium and the left ventricle. It is composed of two cusps of endothelium and resembles a bishop's mitre.

The cusps of these valves are held in place by thin chords, the *chordae tendinae.* These are anchored to projections from the muscular wall called *papillary muscles* (Figure 1.3).

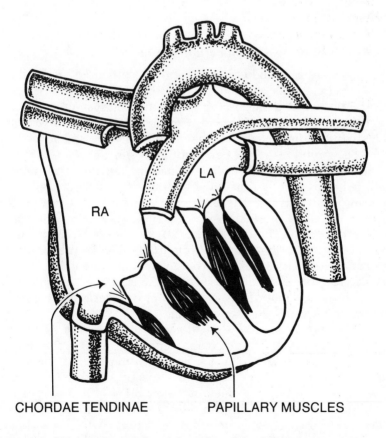

CHORDAE TENDINAE   PAPILLARY MUSCLES

Figure 1.3. Abbreviations: RA = right atrium; LA = left atrium.

The Semilunar Valves are half-moon shaped flaps preventing blood from flowing back into the ventricles (Figure 1.2). The *pulmonary semilunar valve* lies between the pulmonary artery and the right ventricle; the *aortic semilunar valve* lies between the aorta and the left ventricle.

The Fuel Delivery System (Coronary Circulation)

The coronary arteries are the major conduit vessels for oxygenated blood to the heart pump and conduction system. These arteries (right and left) (Figure 1.4) arise from the aorta just above the aortic valve, encircle the heart and penetrate the myocardium. Coronary blood flow may increase or decrease depending on metabolic demands and nervous innervation which may dilate or constrict the vessels.

The Electrical System (Conduction System)

The cardiac conduction system is composed of modified cardiac muscle cells characterized by the ability to conduct electrical impulses. The purpose of the conduction system is to modulate the rate of contraction and to enable the atria and ventricles to contract at the *same rate* rather than separately and at different rates. The structures of the conduction system are:

Sinoatrial node (SA node), or pacemaker, is a small knot of modified heart muscle situated at the junction of the superior vena cava and right atrium. The SA node initiates each heart beat. It initiates impulses approximately 72 times per minute to cause atrial contraction. The determinate of the rate of firing of the SA node are three: 1) *Its inherent automaticity*, i.e., its propensity for automatic depolarization, an event which is caused by shifts in electrolytes through its cell surface; 2) *vagal nerve stimulation* which slows the rate of firing; and 3) *sympathetic nerve stimulation* which increases the rate of firing.

Atrioventricular node (AV node or AV junction) located in the lower aspect of the interarterial septum. The AV node receives electrical impulses from the SA node. Within the AV node, the impulse is delayed for a fraction of a second while the atria complete their contraction and empty their blood into the ventricle. If the SA node fails to fire, the AV node will generate impulses. It generates only 40 to 50 impulses per minute, which is sufficient to sustain human life with reduced activity. Should the AV node

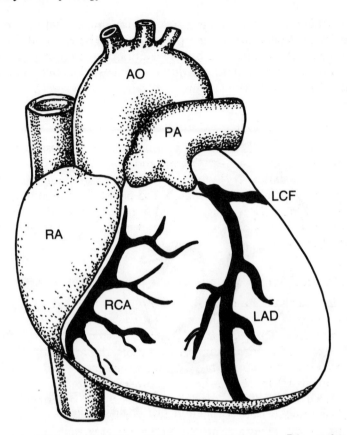

Figure 1.4. Abbreviations: RA = right atrium; AO = aorta; PA = pulmonary artery; RCS = right coronary artery; LAD = left anterior descending; LCF = left circumflex.

also fail, *lower pacemakers* take over the job of impulse formation; they maintain a very low heart rate.

   The bundle of His–Purkinje system is continuous with the AV node. It is composed of specialized cardiac muscle fibers. These fibers pass from the AV node along the upper portion of the inter-ventricular septum then splits into the *right bundle branch* and the *left bundle branch*. The right bundle branch continues under the endocardium toward the apex spreading to all parts of the right ventricle. The left bundle branch penetrates the interventricular septum and comes to lie just under the endocardium of the left ventricle. The left bundle fans out extensively along the endocardial surface of the left ventricle; the major anterior band is called the *anterior fascile;* the posterior band is referred to as the *posterior fascicle.* The terminal conducting fibers or *Purkinje fibers* merge with regular heart muscle to complete the conduction of the electrical impulse (Figure 1.5).

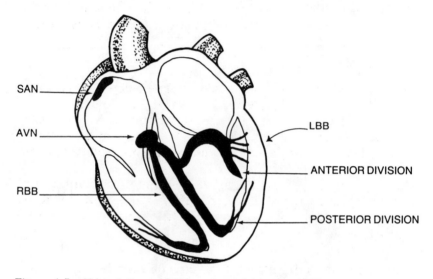

Figure 1.5. Abbreviations: SAN = sinoatrial node; AVN = atrioventricular node; RBB = right bundle branch; LBB = left bundle branch.

NORMAL PHYSIOLOGY OF THE HEART

The heart is essentially a muscle which contracts in response to calcium. Calcium is not itself an activator but initiates the contractile process by releasing an inhibition of contraction by the inhibitory proteins *tropomyosin* and *troponin.*

Cardiac Output and Index

Cardiac output (C.O.) is the volume of blood pumped by the heart each minute and is equivalent to *stroke volume (S.V.)* (i.e., amount of blood ejected with each beat) times *heart rate (H.R.)* (i.e., number of beats per minute).

$$C.O. = S.V. \times H.R.$$

1. *Stroke volume* is approximately 70 ml of blood ejected per heart beat.

2. *Heart rate* is normally 72 beats per minute.

3. *Cardiac output* is, thus, approximately 5,040 ml of blood per minute (i.e., 70 x 72).

The cardiac index is the cardiac output divided by body surface area. Therefore, the cardiac index describes the cardiac output in terms of liters/minute/square meter of body surface.

Cardiac Cycle

One cardiac cycle is equivalent to one complete heart beat, lasting approximately 0.8 seconds. It consists of two parts:

1. *Systole* or contraction of both atria and then both ventricles; systole is initiated by release of an impulse from the SA node.

2. *Diastole*, or relaxation of both atria and then both ventricles.

A cardiac cycle is illustrated in Figure 1.6 starting with diastole, relaxation and filling of the ventricle, going through systole to another following diastole. The arrows demonstrate the direction of blood flow.

Determinants of Performance of the Intact Ventricles

There are four major determinants of performance of the heart: preload, afterload, contractile state, and heart rate.

Preload

The capacity of the intact heart to vary its force of contraction on a beat-to-beat basis in order to meet varying demands is a function of the initial length of the muscle, that which occurs at the end of the diastole. This is called *preload*, or the load at the end of the diastole or the beginning of systole. As this volume of the heart is increased, by increasing venous return of blood, the systolic stroke volume increases. This constitutes one of the major principles of cardiac function and is referred to as *Starling's Law of the Heart* or the *Frank-Starling Phenomenon.*

Afterload

Afterload is the force against which the ventricle has to eject. The major component of afterload is the resistance in the arterial

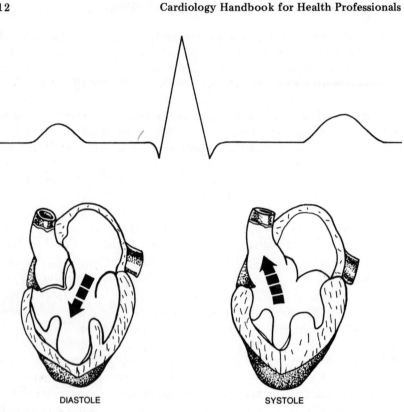

DIASTOLE   SYSTOLE

Figure 1.6.

circulation (systemic vascular resistance). If the ventricle must work against greater resistance, the amount of blood ejected with each contraction (stroke) will decrease.

Contractile State

Contractile state is the performance of the cardiac muscle that is independent of changes resulting from variations in preload or afterload. The basal level of contractility is reduced in myocardial failure. A drug or agent which increases myocardial performance without affecting preload or afterload is referred to as a *positive inotropic agent;* dopamine is an example of such an agent.

Heart Rate

Heart rate at any given instant is determined by 1) *inherent automatic rate of the SA node* plus the relative contribution of 2) the *parasympathetic* and 3) *sympathetic nervous systems*. Parasympathetic influence, which predominates at rest, results in decreased automaticity or slowing of the heart rate and sympathetic influence results in increased automaticity or increase in heart rate. Sympathetic activity predominates during exercise. 4) A fourth determinant of heart rate is the *extrinsic humoral influence* mediated by circulating catecholamines. Administration of certain catecholamine-like drugs, such as theophylline, used in the treatment of asthma, will result in an increase in heart rate similar to the response to the sympathetic nervous system.

Neural Control of Heart

The activity of the autonomic nervous system is of crucial importance in the moment-to-moment regulation of heart rate, contractility, and vascular resistance. Thereby, it controls cardiac output, tissue perfusion and arterial pressure.

The *sympathetic* and *parasympathetic* pathways receive both excitatory and inhibitory impulses to the cardiovascular system and eminate from the cardiovascular centers of the brain (the medulla) and the spinal column. *Efferent* (motor) fibers transmit impulses from the cardiac center in the medulla oblongata to the heart. Sympathetic nerves supply all areas of the atria and ventricles; whereas vagal nerve fibers are primarily found in the SA node, atrial muscle fibers and the AV node. Vagal fibers and vagal impulses also extend to both ventricles although their influence is unclear. Sympathetic stimulus of the heart is mediated by the release of the neurohormone, *norepinephrine*, which increases heart rate and strengthens force of contraction. Cardiac parasympathetic impulses are transmitted by *acetyl-choline*, which decreases heart rate and delays conduction through the AV node. Normally the parasympathetic influence is the dominant autonomic influence on the heart rate, whereas sympathetic influence is the normal dominant influence on ventricular function.

The heart also has sensory (afferent) nerve receptors which provide information to the *vasomotor center* of the brain on heart rate, the force of atrial contraction and the degree of atrial filling. The reflex increase in heart rate that results from stimulation of these receptors helps maintain relatively constant cardiac volume during an increase in venous return. These receptors also act as sensors of the fullness of the bloodstream and hence of the blood volume (Figure 1.7).

Other fibers arise from a widespread nerve network present in all chambers of the heart. When activated, they act like arterial baroceptors to continuously inhibit vasomotor centers, which, in turn decrease the sympathetic outflow to the heart and blood vessels and increase vagal outflow to the heart so that the arterial blood pressure decreases.

Finally, there are sensory nerve connections to the spinal cord. The useful function of these receptors is unknown. It is generally accepted that some are essential to the perception of cardiac pain.

The Peripheral Vascular System

Blood Pressure

This is the pressure exerted by the blood against the walls of the vessels, i.e., arteries, veins, capillaries. The *difference* in blood pressure in arteries, capillaries, and veins or *blood pressure gradient* is the force that enables blood to flow throughout the body. The further blood flows from the heart, the lower the pressure. Pressure is highest in arteries, drops significantly in capillaries, and is almost zero in the great veins. 1) *Systolic pressure* is maximum pressure of the blood exerted against the artery wall when the heart contracts; it is normally 115 to 120 mm Hg. 2) *Diastolic pressure* is the force of blood exerted against the artery walls when the heart is relaxing; it is normally 75–80 mm Hg. 3) *Pulse pressure* is the difference between systolic and diastolic pressures; it is normally 40 mm Hg.

Peripheral Resistance

This is the resistance of the peripheral vascular bed to flow of the blood. This resistance is overcome by the pressure generated by the pumping heart so that blood flows. The blood flow to an organ is determined by the ratio of the *blood pressure gradient* to the resistance to flow offered by the vessel.

Flow = Driving Pressure Gradient / Resistance to Flow

The resistance to flow is determined primarily by the *cross sectional area* of the *arteriolar bed.* This relationship is described by Poiseuille's law that indicates that blood flow is proportional

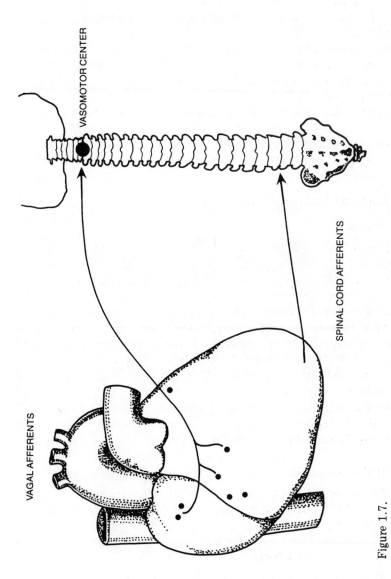

Figure 1.7.

to the fourth power of the radius. Intrinsic humoral and neural influences regulate the vasomotor tone which determines adjustments of the arteriolar bed and consequent flow. The local control of vasomotor tone of the arterioles principally is achieved by *vasodilation*, produced by *metabolic products* and anoxia. The cerebral circulation is particularly sensitive to changes in carbon dioxide tension, while the coronary and skeletal muscle beds adjust to alteration in oxygen tension of the blood. The resistance of the arterioles is also regulated by *sympathetic vasoconstriction*. Vasoconstriction is produced by augmentation of reflex sympathetic nervous activity, and vasodilation occurs as a result of increased local metabolic vasodilator influences and decreased sympathetic vasoconstrictor impulses. In the peripheral vascular beds, receptors for the adrenergic nervouc system, are separated into two types: activation of the *alpha* adrenergic receptors results in arteriole constriction, while activation of the *beta* adrenergic receptors induces arteriolar dilatation.

    Table 1.1 is a schema of interaction between the various components that regulate cardiac activity.

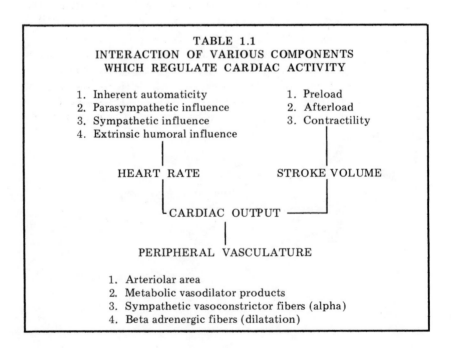

TABLE 1.1
INTERACTION OF VARIOUS COMPONENTS
WHICH REGULATE CARDIAC ACTIVITY

1. Inherent automaticity   1. Preload
2. Parasympathetic influence   2. Afterload
3. Sympathetic influence   3. Contractility
4. Extrinsic humoral influence

HEART RATE   STROKE VOLUME

CARDIAC OUTPUT

PERIPHERAL VASCULATURE

1. Arteriolar area
2. Metabolic vasodilator products
3. Sympathetic vasoconstrictor fibers (alpha)
4. Beta adrenergic fibers (dilatation)

Cardiac Responses During Exertion

The traditional explanation for the increase in cardiac output during exercise is a simultaneous increase in both *heart rate* and *stroke volume*, however, two other considerations must be taken into account before predicting what determines cardiac output during exercise. These are:

1. *The effect of posture on stroke volume.* If a subject is in a relaxed, recumbent position, the stroke volume is near maximal. If the subject is passively tilted upright or stands relaxed, there is a pronounced fall in stroke volume and a significant decrease in heart size.

If the stroke volume obtained during heavy exercise is compared to the recumbent stroke volume at rest, the increase is slight. If, however, the comparison is made with the value obtained when the subject was standing at rest, the increase in stroke volume with exercise is considerable.

2. *The effect of training.* There is good evidence that stroke volume increases with exercise in well trained athletes. Conditioning appears to enhance the possibility for development of a relatively larger increase in stroke volume. The Frank–Starling effect appears to be the major contributor to this augmented SV; however, some studies have suggested an enhanced contractility state in the trained individual.

Hence, the typical cardiovascular response of the untrained individual to exercise is: 1) an increase in oxygen delivery to the tissues mediated by an increase in heart rate with little change in stroke volume, and 2) an increased oxygen extraction by the tissues. The trained individual adds to this an ability to augment stroke volume.

Chapter 2

TOOLS USED IN THE DIAGNOSIS
OF CARDIOVASCULAR DISEASE

ELECTROCARDIOGRAPHY

Technical Aspects

An electrocardiograph is based upon the principle of the *string galvanometer*, described by Einthoven in 1902. Direct writing electrocardiographs are used almost exclusively today but the principles expounded by Einthoven still hold in understanding the basic concepts. The string galvanometer consists of a strong electromagnet, between the poles of which is suspended a string made of a quartz glass fiber about the diameter of a red blood cell (7.8 micron). The fiber is coated with platinum or silver to permit the transmission of an electric current (Figure 2.1). The *magnetic*

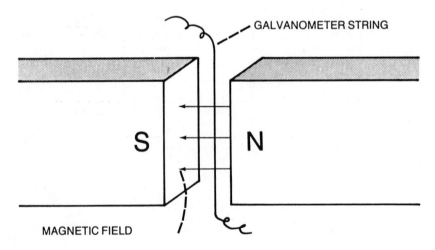

Figure 2.1.

field is a field of constant force set up by the electromagnet. The force runs from the north (N) to the south (S) pole of the magnet. Electric current associated with activity of the heart, conducted through the string, creates another field of force which runs around the long axis of the string and travels either in a clockwise or counterclockwise direction as viewed from one end of the string, depending upon the direction of flow of current in the string. This field around the string is a *magnetic field of variable force*, the magnitude of which depends upon the magnitude of the current flowing through the string. It is the interaction of these two fields with each other that causes movement of the string.

By means of a system of lenses similar to those used in a microscope, the shadow of the string is focused on the slit of a camera in which photographic paper moves, making it possible to record the deflection of the string.

The time and millimeter lines of the electrocardiogram. Figure 2.2 is an enlargement of the horizontal and vertical lines inscribed on the electrocardiogram. The former are 1 mm apart

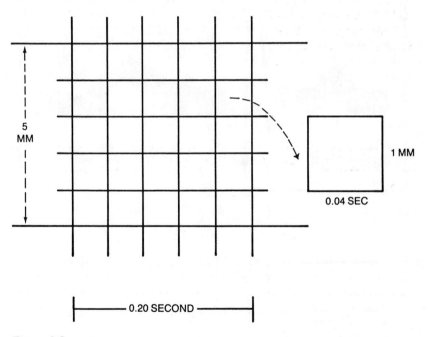

Figure 2.2.

and represent 0.1 millivolt (110 microvolts) when the electrocardiogram is properly standardized. The vertical lines are time lines,
separated from each other by an interval of 0.04 second.

The Normal Electrocardiogram

The typical electrocardiogram consists of a series of deflections designated by Einthoven as the *P wave*, the *QRS complex*,
the *T wave* and the *U wave* (Figure 2.3).

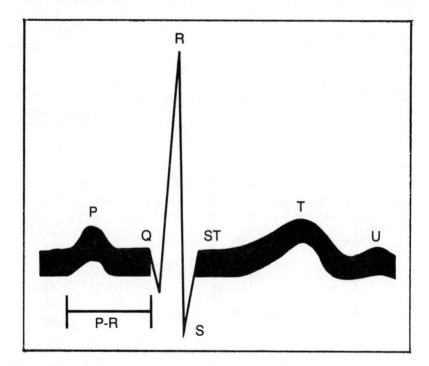

Figure 2.3.

The *P wave* represents the depolarization wave of atrial musculature which spreads rapidly from the sinoatrial (SA) node to
the atrioventricular (AV) node.

The *P–R segment* represents the delay in transmission of the
impulse at the AV node.

The *P–R interval* represents the time required to depolarize the atrial musculature plus the delay in transmission of the impulse through the atrioventricular node to the beginning of ventricular depolarization. The upper limit of normal for the duration of the P-R internal for average cardiac rates in adults is 0.20 second.

The *QRS complex* is the depolarization complex of the ventricular musculature. It consists, usually, of an initial downward deflection, the *Q wave*, an initial upward deflection, the *R wave*, a downward deflection after the R wave, the *S wave*, and a second upward deflection, the second positive deflection or the *R prime (R') wave.* The duration of the QRS is measured in seconds from the beginning of the first wave of the complex to the end of the last wave and does not normally exceed 0.10 second.

The *S-T segment* is the portion of the electrocardiogram between the end of the QRS complex and the beginning of the T wave. It represents the interval of time between the completion of depolarization and the beginning of repolarization of the ventricular musculature.

The *Junction, J point* is the point of junction between the QRS complex and the S-T segment.

The *Q-T interval* is measured in seconds from the beginning of the QRS to the end of the T wave and represents the entire time required for depolarization and repolarization of the ventricular musculature. The upper limit of normal for a heart rate of 70 beats per minute is 0.40 second.

The *T wave* is the wave of ventricular repolarization.

The *U wave* is an "after-potential" wave and is thought to represent His-Purkinje system repolarization.

Classification of Leads

Standard Bipolar Limb Leads

Lead I: Measures the difference in electrical potential between the left arm and right arm.

Lead II: Measures the difference in potential between the left leg and right arm.

Lead III: Measures the difference in potential between the left leg and left arm.

Precordial Leads (V1 through V6)

Electrodes are placed at six different points on the chest wall overlying the heart.

Augmented Unipolar Limb Leads

aVr: Measures electrical potential between the center of the heart and the right arm ("a" stands for augmented, "V" for unipolar, and "r" for right arm).

aVl: Measures electrical potential between the center of the heart and the left arm ("l" stands for left arm).

aVf: Measures electrical potential between the center of the heart and between left leg ("f" stands for foot).

AMBULATORY ELECTROCARDIOGRAPHY

A routine 12-lead ECG takes only a few seconds to obtain, and frequently this is entirely normal even though the patient may be having periodic symptomatic episodes which may be due to abnormalities in the automaticity or rhythm of the heart beat. Dizziness, palpations and black-outs are common manifestations of such cardiac events. Ambulatory (Holter) electrocardiography is a 24-hour recording of continuous ECG rhythm that is accomplished with a portable, lightweight (less than 3 lbs.) battery-powered recorder with miniature amplifiers. It is worn around the waist or carried over the shoulder to facilitate reasonably unencumbered ambulatory activity. A one or two lead system can be used for detecting both rhythm abnormalities and changes in ST-T wave segments. After the recording, the tape is played back by a technician on a scanner in which each QRS complex is superimposed on its predecessor on an oscilliscope at high speed (30-120 times real time). If each QRS has the same configuration, it will appear as a single QRS on the scope. But, if a complex differs from the preceding one the mismatched complex can be identified and recorded on an ECG strip at normal speed. The physician then can conveniently interpret the mounted strips as he would a standard ECG.

EXERCISE STRESS TEST

Since exercise causes the cardiovascular system to operate under stress and many symptoms caused by cardiovascular disease

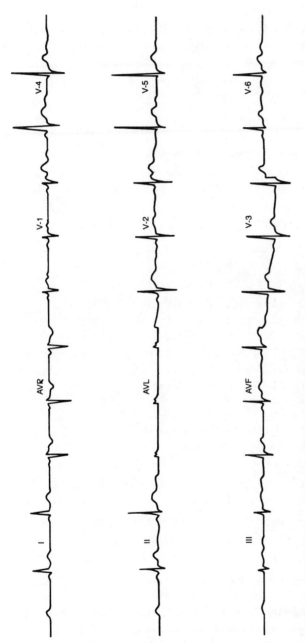

Figure 2.4. Illustrates a normal electrocardiogram in each twelve leads.

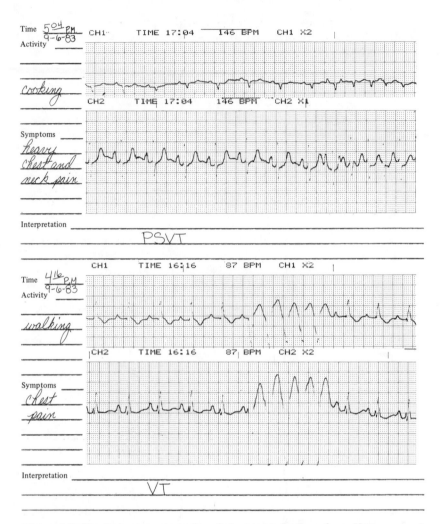

Figure 2.5. Illustrates two examples of abnormal rhythms from Holter recordings.

are brought on by exercise, the exercise stress test is very useful to uncover hidden disease. With proper technique and monitoring equipment, the exercise stress test can be performed safely with the accumulation of much needed information.

Some applications of exercise testing are:
1. Evaluate functional capacity.

2. Assess prognosis and severity of heart disease.
3. Evaluate the effects of treatment.
4. Bring out exercise-related cardiac arrhythmias.
5. Collect baseline data used to prescribe an exercise program.
6. Assess blood pressure response to exercise.
7. Bring out latent evidence of peripheral vascular disease.

There are several exercise protocols which have different workloads at different stages of the test. Either a walking treadmill or a bicycle ergometer is used and changes in the workload are made at regular intervals, usually every 3 minutes, resulting in a progressive rise in oxygen consumption (Table 2.1). After thou-

TABLE 2.1
A TREADMILL EXERCISE TEST PROTOCOL
(Bruce Protocol)

Stage	Speed (MPH)	Elevation	Duration (Minutes)
1	1.7	10%	3
2	2.5	12%	3
3	3.4	14%	3
4	4.2	16%	3
5	5.0	18%	3
6	5.5	20%	3
7	6.0	22%	3

sands of tests, nomograms have been prepared which relate maximal oxygen consumption to age and sex. Any given individual's maximal response at the time of the test can be related to the expected response. If maximal oxygen consumption is not measured, it can be estimated by noting the maximal achievable heart rate and again comparing this to the expected rate for age and sex (Table 2.2).

The widest application of the exercise stress test is in the diagnosis of ischemic heart disease. Ischemia of the cardiac muscle is produced by an imbalance between supply of energy provided by the coronary vessels and demand for oxygen and energy by the working myocardial cells. This imbalance can be precipitated by increasing the myocardial oxygen demand with exercise. Once

TABLE 2.2							
TARGET HEART RATES ON GRADED EXERCISE TEST							
AGE (years)	30	35	40	45	50	55	60
Predicted maximal heart rate (men)	193	191	189	187	184	182	180
Predicted maximal heart rate (women)	190	185	181	177	172	168	163

ischemia develops, the myocardial cell fails to function properly, and one of the results of this dysfunction is manifest in changes in the electrocardiogram, notably the repolarization wave (ST-T segment). The most ominous type of ST segment response on exercise is illustrated in B of Figure 2.6, the down–sloping ST segment. This type of response to exercise has a high degree of predictability for the presence of significant disease of the coronary arteries.

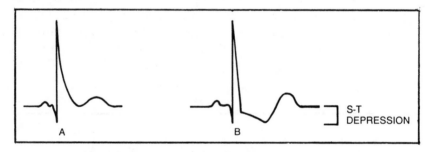

Figure 2.6.

Adequate monitoring and supervision of stress tests includes continuous multiple lead electrocardiography, and blood pressure measurement every two to three minutes. Exercise induced hypotension suggests impaired systolic performance of the ventricle and is a significant finding.

The technician should be trained in resuscitative techniques. Resuscitative equipment, including a defibrillator, should be closely available. Physician supervision is important in order to determine when the test is diagnostic and to terminate the test at the first sign of an adverse response.

CARDIAC IMAGING (NUCLEAR CARDIOLOGY)

Techniques of cardiac imaging using radiopharmaceuticals have proved very useful in both the diagnosis and functional assessment of heart disease. Imaging of the heart is accomplished by injecting a radiopharmaceutical which is tagged to a blood element such as the red cell or one which has avidity for some component of the heart muscle.

Technetium 99M Stannous Pyrophosphate (Tc99M–PYP)

Technetium 99M stannous pyrophosphate (Tc99M-PYP) imaging of acute myocardial infarction was one of the earliest cardiac imaging techniques to gain wide acceptance. After an acute myocardial infarction, calcium is deposited in the region of the infarct and pyrophosphate accumulation in the site is temporarily related to the calcium deposition.

Figure 2.7 illustrates an image of Tc99M-PYP uptake in an area of the heart corresponding to an acute myocardial infarct.

Pyrophosphate imaging is approximately 89% sensitive for the detection of myocardial infarction and 86% specific, meaning that it will usually rule out an infarction in a normal heart (1).

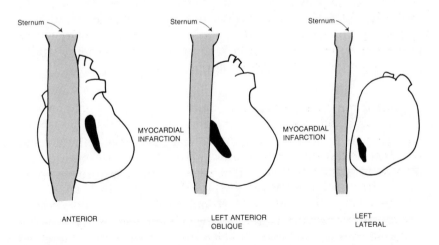

Figure 2.7.

Thallium 201 Exercise Perfusion

Thallium 201 exercise perfusion has proven useful to detect myocardial perfusion abnormalities and has greatly increased the sensitivity of exercise stress testing. Regional coronary blood flow is generally normal and near normal at rest. With exercise an imbalance between myocardial oxygen supply and demand develops. Tl-201 is injected during a period of exercise stress when the heterogeneity of regional myocardial blood flow is maximal. Thallium 201 is a myocardial perfusion agent, its distribution determined by regional myocardial perfusion and cellular viability. Myocardial cells actually take up Tl-201. Poorly perfused zones, i.e., from decreased coronary perfusion, do not accumulate as much tracer as normal zones. During the recovery period, following exercise, there is efflux of Thallium from the well-perfused nonischemic zones and uptake by previously ischemic zones. This equilibration of Tl-201 actively has been termed "redistribution." Images are obtained immediately after exercise and 2-4 hours later at the time of redistribution. Comparison of the two images allows the detection of relative hypoperfusion associated with the transient ischemia of exercise. Definite perfusion abnormalities that are present at the exercise study but not at redistribution or rest are indicative of transient myocardial ischemia. Perfusion defects present at exercise that are unchanged at redistribution are most consistent with previous myocardial infarction.

Overall sensitivity of Tl-201 stress test has been reported to be 75-85%, i.e., it will detect perfusion abnormalities in 75-85% of people subsequently shown to have significant coronary artery disease. It is approximately 90% specific, i.e., it rules out significant coronary disease in 90% of normal hearts.

Nuclide Angiography

Nuclide angiography consists of imaging cardiac structure and function as the radioactive bolus passes through the heart. This requires a radioactive agent that does not leak into surrounding tissues from the cardiac chambers. Technetium labeled red cells stay in the cardiovascular system and images may be obtained as the tracer passes through the heart ("first-pass study") or be triggered at specific times in the cardiac cycle ("multiple gated acquisition" = "MUGA"). The gating is achieved by triggering the

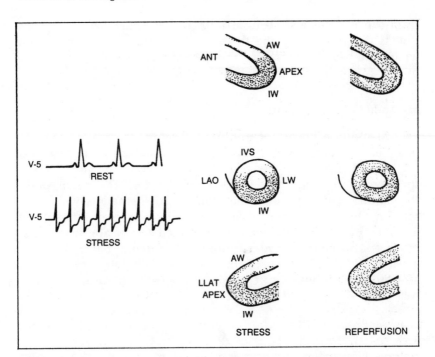

Figure 2.8. Shows rest and stress electrocardiograms and Tl-201 scintigrams. Abbreviations: ANT = anterior; AW = anterior wall; IW = inferior wall; IVS = interventricular septum; LAO = left anterior oblique; LW = lateral wall; LLAT = left lateral.

image to be taken at specific times in the electrocardiographic cycle, times which correspond to specific mechanical activity, e.g., end-diastole or end-systole.

These studies have many uses including evaluation of intra-cardiac shunts in congenital heart disease, regional wall motion or response to exercise in coronary artery disease, or quantitation of the degree of valvular regurgitation.

ECHOCARDIOGRAPHY

Pulsed ultrasound (echocardiography) utilizes sound waves in the range of 1 to 7 million cycles/second or 1 to 7 megaHertz (MHz). Ultrasound creates an image by reflecting the sound waves from the surfaces and structures of the heart; the degree of reflection is determined by the density of the object and the angle at which the beam strikes, the more perpendicular the beam is to the object, the higher the percentage of reflected energy.

M-Mode Echocardiography

M-mode echocardiography ("M" refers to motion) or single plane echocardiography is the first ultrasound method introduced for clinical diagnosis. The transducer is placed on the surface of the chest, alongside the left sternal border. The beam passes through a small portion of the right ventricle, the interventricular septum, the left ventricular cavity and the posterior left ventricular wall (Figure 2.9). When these reflected echoes are written on a moving strip chart recorder calibrated for depth and moving at a given rate (25-100 cm/sec), one may accurately determine both size and rate of motion of the various cardiac structures.

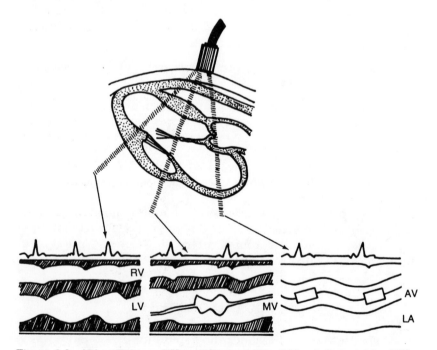

Figure 2.9. Abbreviations: RV = right ventricle; LV = left ventricle; MV = mitral valve; AV = aortic valve; LA = left atrium.

M-mode echocardiography is very valuable in determining single dimensional changes in chamber size and quantitating valve motion during various portions of the cardiac cycle. The technique has proven especially useful in the diagnosis of valvular heart disease.

Two-Dimensional Echocardiography

Two-dimensional echocardiography (cross-section echo; real time echo) is a significant advance over M-mode echo especially where volumes of the ventricular cavity and segmental motion of the ventricular walls are required. This is accomplished by either mechanically sweeping the transducer through an arc thus covering a larger area of the heart, then reconstructing by computer the samples into a 2-dimensional image (*sector scanner*), or by so-called *phased array* where multiple ultrasonic elements are utilized to make up the beam. Figure 2.10 shows several of the cross-sectional images of the heart which may be obtained. 2-D echo has proven valuable in the quantification of myocardial function as well as in assessing the significance of valvular heart disease.

CARDIAC DOPPLER

According to the Doppler principle, when an ultrasonic wave is reflected from a moving object, the frequency of the reflected ultrasound is altered, and the difference in frequency between the

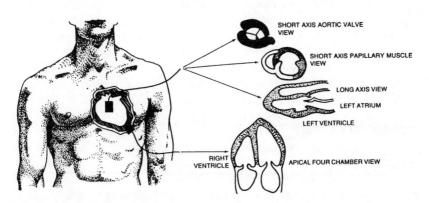

Figure 2.10. 2-D Echo.

ultrasound emitted and that received depends on the velocity of the reflecting interface and the angle at which the beam strikes the object. This change in frequency is referred to as the Doppler shift. Doppler ultrasound is used most often to examine the velocity of blood flow, the ultrasonic energy being reflected by the red blood cells. The technique has proved useful in evaluating blood flow in superficial arteries and veins and to detect obstruction in peripheral arteries.

In combination with two–dimensional echo, pulsed ultrasound has been utilized to determine the velocity of blood flow in certain areas of the heart. This allows the determination of aortic blood flow and flow around the cardiac valves thereby providing information regarding a cardiac output, and valvular function. Figure 2.11 illustrates a Doppler echocardiographic study with mitral regurgitation.

CARDIAC CATHETERIZATION

Cardiac catheterization, the major "invasive" technique of evaluating heart structure and function, consists of passing small catheters from peripheral arteries and veins to the central circulation to measure pressures and flow rates and to inject radiocontrast agents to visualize the chambers and vessels.

Pressures are recorded by attaching the fluid–filled catheters to external pressure transducers which record a change in electrical resistance.

Figure 2.12 illustrates intracardiac pressure waveforms. The right atrial pressure waveform consists of two major positive deflections — the "a" and the "v" waves. The "a" wave is due to atrial systole and the "v" wave is due to ventricular systole. Each is followed by a descent, the "x" and "y" descent, respectively. An additional small wave, the "c" wave, is coincident with tricuspid valve closure.

The diastolic phase of the right ventricular pressure curve consists of a *rapid filling wave (RF)*, during which 60% of ventricular filling occurs, a *slow filling wave (SF)* and an *a wave* of atrial systole.

Pulmonary artery pressure waveforms consist of a systolic pressure, followed by the *incisura (I)* of pulmonic valve closure, then end–diastolic pulmonary artery pressure (ed).

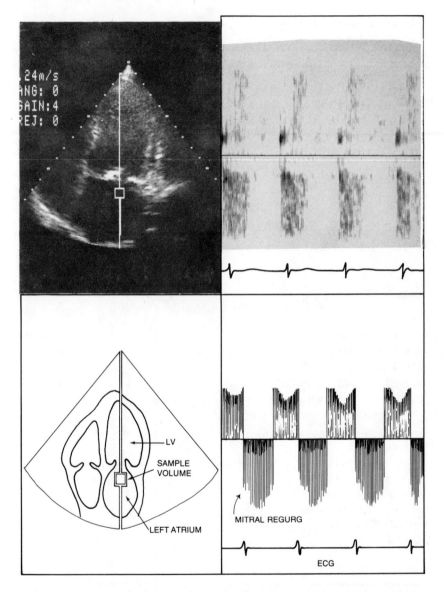

Figure 2.11. Echo–Doppler sample taken from the left atrium showing flow back into the left atrium in systole (Mitral Regurg = mitral regurgitation).

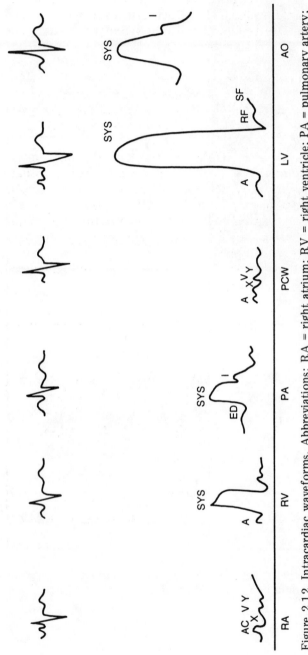

Figure 2.12. Intracardiac waveforms. Abbreviations: RA = right atrium; RV = right ventricle; PA = pulmonary artery; PCW = pulmonary capillary wedge; LV = left ventricle; AO = aorta; SYS = systole; ED = end–diastole.

Pulmonary artery wedge pressure waveform is similar to the right atrial pressure waveform. It reflects left atrial pressure, and in the normal pulmonary circulation of low vascular resistance, the pulmonary artery flow is diminished at end–diastole, so that end-diastolic pulmonary artery and mean pulmonary artery wedge pressures are approximately equal.

Left ventricle waveform components are the peak systolic pressure (Sys), the rapid filling (RF) and slow filling (SF) waves and atrial wave (a) of diastolic filling and the end–diastolic pressure (ed).

Table 2.3 shows the range of normal hemodynamic values.

Coronary arteriography is an invaluable technique for visualization of the coronary vasculature in patients with atherosclerotic coronary vascular disease. It is performed by passing specially designed catheters to the coronary ostia and injecting radiopaque contrast in the vessels while intravascular pressure is carefully monitored.

Figure 2.13A illustrates a right coronary arteriogram and 2.13B a left coronary arteriogram.

TABLE 2.3
RANGE OF NORMAL RESTING HEMODYNAMIC VALUES

Pressure	Systolic	End–Diastolic	Mean
Right atrium			0 to 8
Right ventricle	15 to 30	0 to 8	
Pulmonary artery	15 to 30	3 to 12	9 to 16
Pulmonary capillary wedge			1 to 12
Left ventricle	100 to 140	3 to 12	
Aorta	100 to 140	60 to 90	70 to 105
Cardiac Output Index	2.5 to 4.2 liters/minute		

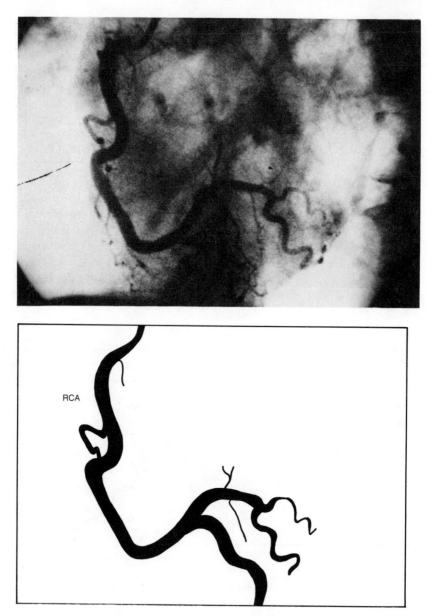

Figure 2.13A. Abbreviation: RCA = right coronary artery

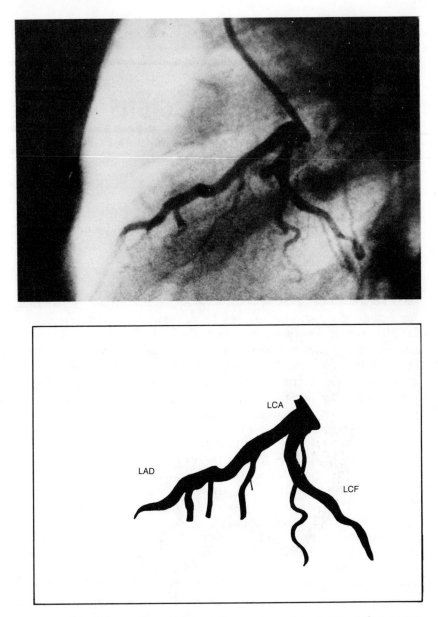

Figure 2.13B. Abbreviations: LCA = left coronary artery; LAD = left anterior descending; LCF = left circumflex.

Chapter 3

SYMPTOMS AND SIGNS OF CARDIOVASCULAR DISEASE

SYMPTOMS OF CARDIOVASCULAR DISEASE

There are four major groups of symptoms which may point to cardiovascular disease: dyspnea, chest pain, palpitation and peripheral edema.

Dyspnea

Dyspnea or shortness of breath (SOB) on exertion. It is important to determine how severe this symptom is by asking how far the patient can walk before becoming SOB. Dypsnea can be caused by pulmonary disease as well as heart disease, and at times it is difficult to make the distinction. Features which suggest pulmonary disease are: a history of asthma or associated wheezing, more difficulty breathing out (expiring) than in (inspiring) and chronic cough with sputum production.

Orthopnea is another symptom associated with dyspnea and consists of dyspnea in the supine position but relief of the symptoms on sitting up. This frequently occurs on going to bed at night when lying down mobilizes the blood which had previously been pooled in the extremities and results in increased blood return to the heart. The patient will often have to raise his head on two or more pillows to sleep comfortably.

Another closely related symptom is *paroxysmal nocturnal dyspnea* which consists of the patient awakening in the night short of breath and being forced to sit up to recover his breath. This is also caused by mobilization of pooled blood from the extremities to the heart, raising pressure in the heart and resulting in dyspnea.

Chest Pain

Chest pain of heart disease (angina pectoris) is classically reported as a tight, pressure–like or squeezing sensation and usually occurs in the left precordium, at mid-sternum and may radiate to the left arm, shoulder, neck or jaw. This is the classic description; however, exceptions to this description can occur including description of the pain as knife-like, dull, or aching and radiation to the back or epigastrium.

The angina is classically brought on by exertion, emotion or extreme anxiety and normally does not last longer than 20 minutes at a time without relief. Angina may occur at rest, and if this variety of the symptom is reported, it should be recognized as a high risk situation warranting prompt attention to prevent progression to a myocardial infarction.

Angina is frequently associated with other symptoms such as dyspnea and heavy perspiration (diaphoresis).

Palpitation

Palpitation is the sensation of the heart skipping a beat or beating too fast. Sensations of a sudden fullness in the throat, a "thump" in the chest or a sudden pounding in the chest are associated with tachycardias and bradycardias. The most common symptom is caused by a single extra systole which occurs early in the cardiac cycle and does not produce a sensation. The following beat, however, is potentiated (post-estrasystolic potentiation), and the individual will feel this augmented contractility.

Dizziness and actual loss of consciousness, *syncope* may be associated with heart rhythm disturbances including bradycardias and tachycardias. Before dizziness or syncope occurs, it usually requires rates as low as 40 beats per minute or as fast as 160 beats per minute.

Peripehral Edema

Peripheral edema may be caused by heart failure where the heart is incapable of pumping adequately and perfusing the body's organs. This is recognized by the kidneys as a sign of decreased blood volume so salt and water are retained, thereby leading to an increase in blood volume and edema.

The edema is usually most easily detected on the anterior surface of the tibial bones (pretibial edema). If the patient has been at bed rest for long periods of time, the edema takes a dependent position and may be found over the sacrum and buttocks.

There are other causes for peripheral edema including renal disease, hormonal disturbances, liver disease or obstruction to veins and lymphatics.

The following is a *functional classification* of symptoms in heart disease:

Class 1. Asymptomatic
Class 2. Symptoms on ordinary exertion
Class 3. Symptoms on less than ordinary exertion
Class 4. Symptoms at rest

SIGNS OF CARDIOVASCULAR DISEASE

Peripheral Signs

Peripheral signs of cardiovascular disease which should be searched for include:

Hemorrhages and petechiae on conjunctive of eyes due to bacterial endocarditis.

Thick yellow *arcus* around the iris may indicate hypercholesterolemia.

Retinal abnormalities in hypertension are:

Grade 1: Generalized attenuation of arterial calibre
Grade 2: Focal constriction
Grade 3: Hemorrhages and exudates
Grade 4: Papilledema

Retinal abnormalities in arteriosclerosis are:

Grade 1: Light reflex has increased width
Grade 2: Crossing defects (arterio–venous nicking)
Grade 3: Copper-wire arteries
Grade 4: Silver-wire arteries

Xanthelasma of the eyes may be associated with hypercholesterolemia.

Blue sclerae of the eyes may be associated with osteogenesis imperfecta, Marfan's syndrome of Ehlers–Danlos syndrome, all of which may have associated cardiac abnormalities.

Xanthomas of the skin may be associated with hypercholesterolemia.

Peripheral cyanosis may be seen in such areas as nail bed, nose, cheeks, earlobe and outer surface of the lips and is associated with congenital heart disease with shunting of unoxygenated blood into the systemic circulation.

Clubbing of the nail beds of the fingers and toes may be found in congenital heart disease and is commonly associated with cyanosis.

Peripheral Pulses

Peripheral pulses which should be palpated include the carotids, brachials, radials, femorals, dorsalis pedis and posterior tibials. The pulses should be palpated for the *rate of rise*. The normal rapid rate of rise is felt as a tapping quality while the slow rate of rise is felt like a slow roll.

The slow rising pulse may be a clue to the presence of severe *aortic stenosis*. This slowly rising pulse has also been called an *anacrotic pulse, pulsus parvus,* or *plateau pulse.*

Very rapid rates of rise of pulse may be found in:
  mitral regurgitation
  ventricular septal defect
  hypertrophic subaortic stenosis (IHSS)
  patent ductus arteriosis
  coarction of the aorta (if palpate arteries proximal to the
        coarctation)
  anemia
  thyrotoxicosis
  pregnancy
  aortic regurgitation

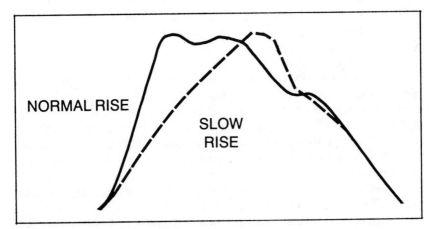

Figure 3.1. Carotid pulse tracing.

Some conditions will result in a *double humped pulse*. Hypertrophic subaortic stenosis (IHSS) will present a "spike and dome" pulse (A in Figure 3.2).

Mitral regurgitation may result in a *dicrotic pulse* where the ejection of blood from the ventricle is shortened and there is a large wave early in diastole (B in Figure 3.2).

The *bisferiens pulse* (C in Figure 3.2) is a double peaked pulse and may be caused by a combination of aortic stenosis and regurgitation.

Blood Pressure

Blood pressure is measured in the arms and legs with a sphygmomanometer and a stethescope. The *Korotkoff sounds* are heard as the artery is auscultated while the pressure in the cuff is released. The onset of the sound indicates *systolic blood pressure*. The point where the Korotkoff sound disappear is the *diastolic blood pressure*.

Blood pressure should be taken in both arms in the supine and standing positions and in the legs if palpation of the arteries has suggested an obstruction.

Other abnormalities of blood pressure include: 1) *Pulsus alternans* which is an alternating fluctuation in pulse pressure and is associated with severe left ventricular dysfunction. 2) *Pulsus paradoxus* which is a decrease of at least 10 mm Hg in systolic blood pressure on inspiration and is associated with pericardial effusion with tamponade or bronchospastic lung disease.

Venous Pressure

The venous pressure is the pressure in the peripheral veins, which is essentially the same as right atrial pressure. It may be estimated by examining the internal jugular vein at the neck. With the patient sitting at a 45 degree angle, the top of the internal jugular vein column is identified, and the height above the sternal angle (where the 2nd rib joins the sternum) is measured. This should not be greater than 4.5 cm above this angle. If it is higher, this suggests increased venous pressure and elevated filling pressure of the right atrium.

Figure 3.3 illustrates the normal jugular venous wave. The major waves are the *A wave* produced by atrial contraction, the

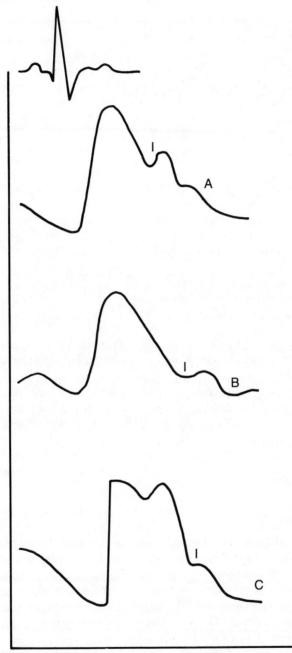

Figure 3.2. Abbreviation: I = incisura.

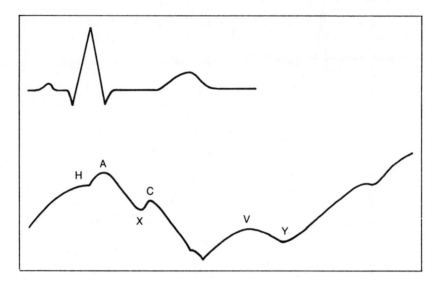

Figure 3.3. Jugular venous pulse tracing.

C wave produced by a fusion of tricuspid valve bulging plus carotid artery artifact, and *V wave* produced by right atrial filling during systole.

Abnormalities of these waves include: 1) *Large A wave* in obstruction to right atrial outflow as in tricuspid stenosis or right atrial myxoma, or stiff (poorly compliant) right ventricle as in pulmonary hypertension or pulmonic stenosis. 2) *Large V wave* in tricuspid regurgitation, high venous pressure in congestive heart failure, or loss of compliance of right atrium, as in constrictive pericarditis.

Auscultation of the Heart

Auscultation of the heart is one of the most important parts of the physical examination. The heart is auscultated with the stethoscope, using the bell for low-frequency sounds and the diaphragm for high-frequency sounds. The left precordium is auscultated at the apex of the heart (about the fifth intercostal space and midclavicular line — also called the *mitral area*), at the lower left sternal border (*area of the tricuspid valve*), upper left sternal border (*area of the pulmonic valve*), and upper right sternal border (*aortic valve area*).

Figure 3.4 illustrates the normal heart sounds at several areas. *Physiologic splitting of the second heart sound* can be detected at the pulmonic area. This refers to the widening of the separation of the aortic and pulmonic closure sound on inspiration. This splitting is due to a decrease in pulmonary vascular compliance on inspiration and consequent delayed closure of the pulmonic valve.

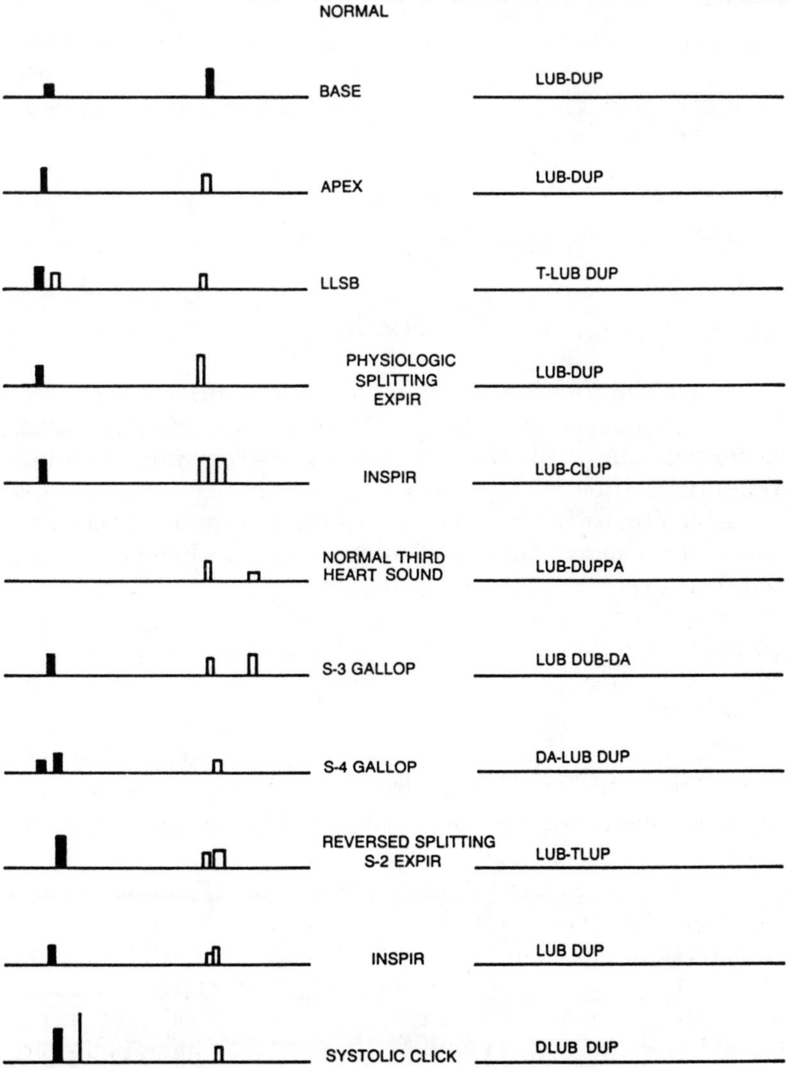

Figure 3.4.

Some abnormal sounds are also illustrated in Figure 3.4. *Gallop sounds* are ventricular filling sounds and may be of right ventricular or left ventricular origin. Respiratory variation, i.e., an increase in intensity during inspiration, marks the sound as of right-sided origin. The S3 gallop occurs in *volume overload* of the ventricle and the S4 gallop signifies *pressure overload* of the ventricle.

Reversed (paradoxical) splitting of the second heart sound may occur in complete left bundle branch block (due to delayed activation of the left ventricle) or any other cause for prolonged left ventricular ejection (severe systemic hypertension or severe aortic valve stenosis).

Systolic ejection clicks may be heard in pulmonic or aortic valvular stenosis. *Non-clicking systolic clicks* may occur with the mitral valve prolapsing syndrome.

MURMURS

A heart murmur is the sound made from turbulence in blood flow. It can be caused when the blood encounters a narrowing in the flow channel. This results in increased velocity at the point of narrowing, setting up turbulence and the generation of a sound. This is similar to the sound from a river as it passes from a wide channel to a narrow rapids. Murmurs occur either in systole of diastole.

Systolic Murmurs

Ejection Type

The ejection type murmur is that produced when blood is being ejected across a narrowed orifice such as *aortic valve stenosis*, or *pulmonic stenosis*. It may be diagrammed as:

"La-raAh-d"

It has a "diamond shaped" quality indicating that the blood flow rises to a peak then tapers off. This murmur is usually low pitched and harsh and best heard with the bell of the stethoscope. The aortic murmur is heard best at the aortic area and the pulmonic murmur best at the pulmonic area.

Regurgitant Type

This murmur is caused by the regurgitation of blood from a high pressure chamber (ventricle) to a relatively low pressure chamber (atrium or, in a VSD, the lower pressure right ventricle). Examples are *mitral regurgitation* or *ventricular septal defect (VSD)*. It may be diagrammed as:

"Laooshdt"

The intensity of the murmur is about the same throughout systole, since the regurgitation begins immediately at the beginning of systole, because the flow from the high pressure area to the low pressure area begins at the beginning of systole and does not have to reach a peak velocity in order to overcome a high resistance. The murmur has a high frequency and best heard with the diaphragm of the stethoscope.

The murmur of mitral regurgitation is heard best at the apex (mitral region) and frequently radiates to the axilla. The murmur of tricuspid regurgitation is heard best at the tricuspid area and increases in intensity on inspiration (as do all sounds, gallops and murmurs of right–sided origin). The murmur of ventricular septal defect (VSD) is best heard along the left sternal border.

Other Systole Murmurs

Atrial septal defect (ASD) results in a murmur of pulmonic valve origin. It is an ejection type murmur heard at the pulmonic area. It is classically associated with *fixed split second heart sound,* i.e., the aortic and pulmonic components of the second heart sound are widely split and remain so during inspiration and expiration. It may be diagrammed as:

"lub-sshhss-cll-ub"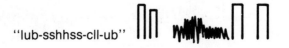

The murmur of *Hypertrophy Cardiomyopathy (Idiopathic Hypertrophic Subaortic Stenosis)* is caused by a dynamic obstruction to left ventricular outflow. Its character is somewhere between that of aortic valvular stenosis and mitral regurgitation and is best heard at the lower left sternal border and apex. The major feature of this murmur is its dynamic nature. Its intensity may be varied by such maneuvers as: valsalva (increase in intensity of murmur), amyl nitrate (increase), standing upright (increase), or squatting (decrease).

Mitral valve prolapse (MVP) is caused by buckling (prolapse) of the mitral valve back into the left atrium during systole. It is classically introduced by a "click" or snapping sound which is thought to be secondary to the sudden tensing of the chordae. The click and murmur may be diagrammed as:

"La-kissdt"

This is also a dynamic murmur and its intensity and timing is affected by any maneuver which changes ventricular volume which determines the tautness of the chordae. For example: Amyl nitrite decreases ventricular volume and brings the click and murmur earlier in systole; a similar result can be expected on standing; squatting may increase ventricular volume and make the click–murmur occur later in systole or disappear entirely.

Diastolic Murmurs

These murmurs are due to turbulent flow across valves in diastole.

Mitral valvular stenosis is caused by rheumatic fever and results in a low rumbling diastolic murmur caused by blood flowing from the left atrium to the left ventricle. It may be diagrammed as:

"la-da-cra-u-ah-la-da"

sl(ml)

A2
P2
OS   DR   PSM

The murmur may be introduced by an opening snap (O.S.) which is a snapping sound of the diseased valve. The murmur may only be heard by placing the patient in the left lateral position which rotates the heart towards the chest wall. One must use the bell of the stethoscope and place it lightly at the point of maximal apex beat, usually about the 5th intercostal space, just lateral to the mid–clavicular line.

Tricuspid valvular stenosis is more unusual but has the same characteristics as MS and is heard at the tricuspid area.

Aortic valvular regurgitation (AR) is also usually caused by rheumatic fever although other etiologies include syphilis, congenital bicuspid aortic valve, Marfan's syndrome, collagen vascular disease including Reiter's disease and ankylosing spondylitis. It may be diagrammed as:

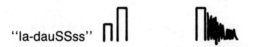

"la-dauSSss"

It consists of a diastolic blow decrescendo (decreasing in intensity) murmur. It may be best heard at the aortic area, or commonly, all along the left sternal border.

Pulmonic valvular insufficiency (pulmonic regurgitation PR) may result from rheumatic heart disease or pulmonary hypertension. It is a very uncommon murmur when present, it is heard best at the upper left sternal border.

Other Murmurs

Patent ductus arteriosis (PDA) between the pulmonary artery and aorta will produce a continuous machinery–like murmur. It may be diagrammed as:

"a-raw-uh-a-raw-a"

Pericarditis will produce a *pericardial friction rub* which classically has 3 components — one long scratchy sound in systole and two scratchy diastolic sounds.

Chapter 4

DISEASES OF THE FUEL SYSTEM OF THE HEART (The Coronary Arteries)

INTRODUCTION

Coronary artery disease is the leading cause of death in men 45-64 years of age in the United States, as well as in most of the western industrialized countries. The major cause of coronary artery disease is atherosclerosis which is found in some degree in the majority of adult men in the U.S. regardless of symptoms. Almost 4,400,000 Americans have a history of angina or myocardial infarction; there are an estimated 1,500,000 heart attacks every year and the death toll from myocardial infarction approaches 350,000 yearly.

The cause of the atherosclerotic lesion is not clearly understood. The atherosclerotic plaque is composed of a complex of lipids (cholesterol and other lipids), fibrous tissue, calcium and smooth muscle cells. The lesions appear to begin to develop at a very early age and slowly increase in size, eventually leading to hemorrhage, ulceration and thrombosis of the artery.

Although the cause of the atherosclerotic plaque is unknown, epidemiologic studies have revealed an association of certain *risk factors* with the development of atherosclerosis. None of these factors are known to actually cause the disease, but their presence in an individual significantly increases the risk of development of the disease.

Table 4.1 lists the possible risk factors for coronary heart disease. Age, sex and family history are immutable factors, the over 40-year-old male with a strong family history being at highest risk. Some associations are stronger than others — hypertension, cigarette smoking, elevated serum cholesterol and low high density lipoprotein being the strongest risks.

Coronary artery disease has four major presentations: angina pectoris, myocardial infarction, congestive heart failure, and sudden cardiac death.

TABLE 4.1
POSSIBLE RISK FACTORS FOR CORONARY ARTERY DISEASE

Immutable:	Age
	Sex
	Family history
Strong:	Hypertension
	Cigarette smoking
	Elevated serum cholesterol
	Low high density lipoprotein (HDL)
Uncertain Importance:	Personality type
	Physical inactivity
Weak:	Heredity, as independent variable
	Obesity, as independent variable
	Diabetes mellitus
Questionable:	Stress
	Serum uric acid
	Soft water
Probably Not:	Serum triglyceride
	Coffee
	Dietary sugar
	Dietary animal protein

ANGINA PECTORIS

Angina pectoris or pain in the chest was first described as a clinical entity by William Heberden in 1768. It is caused by *ischemia* of the myocardial tissues which occurs when the demand for energy exceeds that which the coronary arteries can supply. The characteristics of the chest pain were described in chapter three.

Ischemia occurs when there is an imbalance between demand and supply. The factors which determine coronary oxygen and energy substrate supply are: 1) anatomy (calibre of vessels), 2) autoregulation of vessels, 3) perfusion pressure, and 4) oxygen carrying capacity. The factors which determine myocardial oxygen demand are: 1) contractility, 2) load on the ventricle (preload and afterload), 3) wall thickness, and 4) heart rate. So there are two etiologic types of angina pectoris, that caused by *increased demand* and that caused by *decreased supply*.

Increased Demand Angina Pectoris

Increased demand angina pectoris (Heberden's angina, classic angina) is produced when an increase in myocardial oxygen demand cannot be met because of a fixed coronary blood supply. This is the most common type of angina and is the type usually associated with atherosclerotic plaques of the vessels. When the plaque occludes at least 70% of the lumen of a vessel, then inadequate coronary blood supply will result, and any activity which calls for an increase in demand on the ventricle will result in ischemia.

The usual situations where angina occurs because of an increase in myocardial oxygen demand are:

Exercise: Increases heart rate and blood pressure.

Postprandial: Following a meal, more of the body's blood is shunted to the digestive organs so that any exercise at this time will result in a relatively greater increase in heart rate and blood pressure.

Fear, anxiety, anger: These emotions cause catecholamines to be produced resulting in an increase in heart rate, blood pressure and contractility. This is the mechanism for some types of nocturnal angina including that produced by dreams.

Supine position: Lying down after prolonged standing may cause mobilization of fluids from peripheral tissues to the ventricle increasing preload and, thereby, wall tension.

Figure 4.1 illustrates a frame from the coronary arteriogram of a 39-year-old gambler who related left precordial jaw and arm pain while watching football games on which he had placed bets. A very tight lesion of the left anterior descending coronary artery can be seen.

Decreased Supply Angina Pectoris

Decreased supply angina pectoris (Prinzmetal's angina, reverse angina, variant angina) usually occurs at rest with a cyclic variation during the day. It is caused by spasm of the coronary vessels from unknown causes. Classically the angina begins without an increase in demand, without a rise in blood pressure or heart rate. The ischemia of the ventricle may result in impaired systolic performance of the ventricle resulting in a subsequent drop in blood pressure.

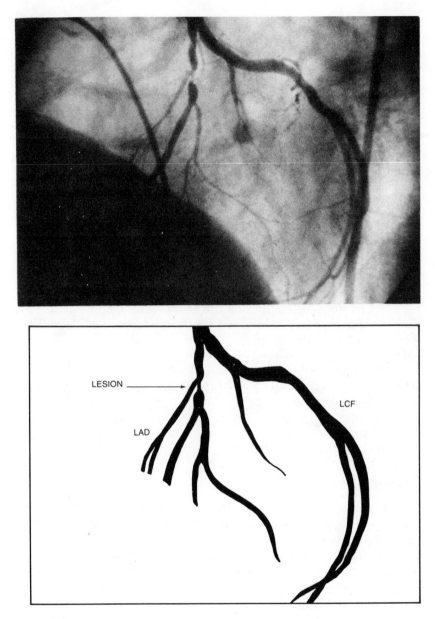

Figure 4.1.

Figure 4.2 shows two frames of a coronary arteriogram from a patient with variant angina. The angina is caused by *spasm* of the coronary vessel and consequent decreased coronary blood supply.

Diangosis of Angina Pectoris

Examination During an Attack

One of the most useful diagnostic techniques for establishing the presence of angina pectoris is the examination of the patient during an attack. Because of ischemia of the heart, several abnormalities may appear which were not present on a prior, angina-free exam, including:

Gallop sound, especially S4

Heart murmurs, especially papillary muscle dysfunction

Paradoxic splitting of S2

Dyskinetic (bulging) left ventricular apex

Hypertension of hypotension and tachycardia

ST-T abnormalities on the electrocardiogram

Increase in diastolic ventricular pressures and decrease in cardiac output.

Exercise Stress Test

Exercise stress test with ECG monitoring is commonly used to increase myocardial oxygen demand and provoke ischemia. This test has been discussed in chapter two. Once the demand is increased with exercise, ST-T abnormalities may appear on the electrocardiogram establishing the diagnosis.

Ergonovine Provocation Test

Ergonovine provocation test is sometimes used to provoke coronary spasm in suspected cases of variant angina. Ergonovine is given intravenously in very small increments until a total upper limit dose is administered or until ECG changes of ischemia occur or coronary spasm are demonstrated on coronary arteriography.

Treatment of Angina Pectoris

Drug Treatment

Table 4.2 shows the major agents which are used to treat angina pectoris. *Nitrates*, the oldest form of treatment, work both

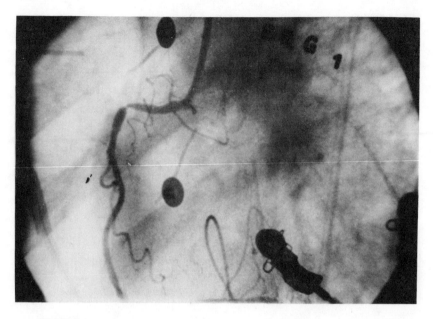

SPASM

RCA

Figure 4.2A. Abbreviation: RCA = right coronary artery.

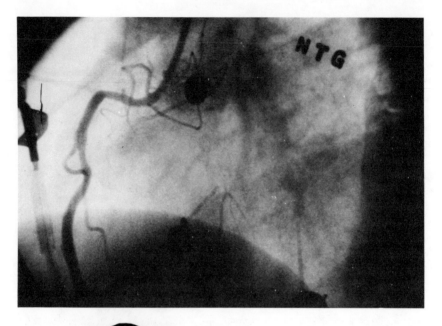

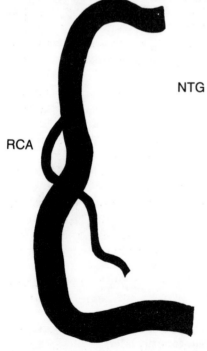

NTG

RCA

Figure 4.2B. Abbreviations: RCA = right coronary artery; NTG = nitroglycerin.

TABLE 4.2
AGENTS USED IN TREATMENT OF ANGINA PECTORIS

	Agent	Effect
Nitrates	nitroglycerin	Dilates arterioles
	isosorbide dinitrate	and veins
	dermal nitroglycerin	Dilates coronary vessels
Beta Blockers	propranolol	Decrease heart rate
	metoprolol	Decrease blood pressure
	nadolol	Decrease ventricular
	atenolol	contractility
	timolol	
	pindolol	
Calcium Channel Blockers	nifedipine	Dilate coroary aa.
	verapamil	Dilate arterioles
	diltiazem	

centrally by producing coronary vasodilatation, and peripherally by dilating the compliance vessels, thereby decreasing the load upon the heart. Arterial blood pressure is decreased also. The potentially adverse effect of nitrates is the increase in heart rate which is produced by reflex baroreceptors in response to the decrease in arterial pressure.

There are currently many different nitrate preparations which provide different sites and rates of absorption: Sublingual — rapid absorption, lasting 2 hours; oral — ½ hour absorption, lasting 4-6 hours; dermal — slow, continuous absorption, lasting 24 hours.

Beta-blockers are used to treat angina pectoris for their ability to decrease heart rate, blood pressure and myocardial contractility. The major adverse effect of these drugs is the increase in end-diastolic volume of the ventricles which may precipitate heart failure in individuals with borderline left ventricular function. Various B-blockers are available with different degrees of cardioselectivity (the ability to block specific cardiac beta receptors) and different durations of action.

In combination with nitrates, B-blockers are potent antianginal agents, each counteracting the adverse effects of the other agent.

The third class of drugs which have proved useful in the treatment of angina pectoris is *calcium channel antagonists*. The calcium channel is the major source of calcium for contraction of smooth muscle of arteries. Blocking this calcium channel will result in peripheral vascular dilatation and dilatation of the coronary vasculature. In addition to increasing coronary blood flow, these agents decrease myocardial oxygen demand by their action on peripheral arteries. The three calcium channel antagonists which are currently available are nifedipine, verapamil and diltiazem.

These three types of antianginal therapy may be used in various combination if careful attention is paid to interacting effects. For example, nitrates and calcium antagonists both produce some degree of hypotension and can be used together if arterial blood pressure is carefully monitored. Calcium antagonists and B-blockers have been found to complement each other in the management of previously refractory angina pectoris.

Percutaneous Transluminal Coronary Angioplasty (PCTA)

Percutaneous transluminal coronary angioplasty (PCTA) has been found to be an important and valuable treatment modality in angina pectoris. The technique consists of threading a very small deflated balloon down the coronary vessel to the region of the previously demonstrated lesion. The balloon is then inflated with high pressure and the lesion is dilated and flattened against the arterial wall. The technique takes special skill and training but in these hands has proven to be very useful in carefully selected cases with resultant decrease in the manifestation of ischemia. Figure 4.3 illustrates the balloon passing a lesion and the resultant dilation of the lesion.

The coronary lesions which are most amenable to PCTA are proximal lesions of single coronary vessels although some success has been achieved against selected multivessel disease.

Coronary Artery Bypass Grafting (CABG)

Coronary artery bypass grafting (CABG) is extremely successful in the management of angina pectoris. The technique consists of implanting a vein from the ascending aorta to the diseased coronary vessel beyond the lesion (Figure 4.4). This significantly increases blood flow to the ischemic region and relieves the angina. The major indication for CABG are: 1) medically intractable angina, i.e., if angina continues despite adequate medical treatment, 2) critical coronary artery lesions, i.e., disease of the left

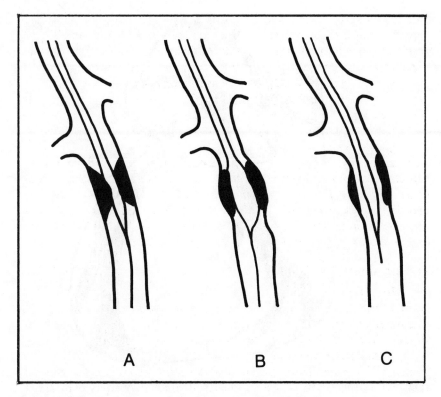

Figure 4.3. Percutaneous transluminal coronary angioplasty.

main coronary artery, disease of the three major coronary arteries (three-vessel disease), or disease of the proximal left anterior descending coronary artery.

MYOCARDIAL INFARCTION

Myocardial infarction (MI) or heart attack is the term used when there is actual death or necrosis of myocardial cells. It may be the end result of progressive angina pectoris, or it may occur suddenly from the sudden occlusion of a coronary vessel.

Causes of Myocardial Infarction

Thrombus on a previously subtotal atherosclerotic lesion. *Embolus* down a coronary vessel. This embolus may originate

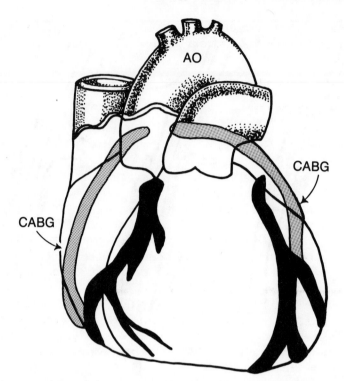

Figure 4.4. Abbreviations: AO = aorta; CABG = coronary artery bypass graft.

from a thrombus in the ventricle or from an endocarditis vegetation on the aortic valve.

Spasm of a coronary vessel may rarely result in necrosis (infarction) of myocardium.

Trauma to the chest wall with involvement of the heart may result in myocardial necrosis similar to MI, without thrombosis of the coronary vessel.

Presentation of an MI most commonly consists of the onset of severe precordial pain, similar to that described in angina pectoris, only more severe. The pain may radiate to the jaw, left or both arms or back. It is usually associated with shortness of breath, sweating and pallor. A ventricular arrhythmia may occur at this time, and the patient may not survive the acute attack unless prompt cardiopulmonary resuscitation is instituted.

In a significant percentage of cases, there is little or no pain (in as many as 25% of MIs). The painless MI is more common in diabetics, who, presumably, have diabetic neuropathy and decreased pain sensations from the heart.

Diagnosis of Myocardial Infarction

Electrocardiography

Myocardial infarction is usually diagnosed by electrocardiography which shows: 1) Q waves, and 2) ST-T abnormalities.

Abnormal Q waves (greater than = .03 sec.) indicate necrosis in the region sampled. Common areas of MI and their ECG abnormalities are illustrated in Figure 4.5.

Initially the ECG has elevated ST-T waves over the infarcted region. Over several days these ST-T abnormalities evolve and return to the baseline. T waves may be inverted at this stage, later to return to normal. If the ST segment remains elevated, this is evidence for the development of an *aneurysm* (a ballooning myocardial wall) in the region of the MI.

Nontransmural Myocardial Infarction (subendocardial MI) is the term used to refer to myocardial necrosis which does not involve the entire wall of the myocardium. This results in ST-T abnormalities which evolve like those of a transmural MI, however Q waves are not present.

Limitations of the ECG: The ECG may not be diagnostic in the presence of myocardial necrosis. There are several reasons for this false negativity, including the infarct may be outside of the sampled region, the infarct may be small and remain undetected and, most commonly, other ECG changes may mask the infarction pattern, especially bundle branch block or ventricular hypertrophy.

Cardiac Enzymes

Cardiac enzymes are extremely useful in the diagnosis of MI. These are proteins which are present in myocardial cells (as well as other tissues) and are spilled into the peripheral circulation when there is injury to the cell wall. Injury to other tissues may also raise these enzymes, but the patterns of rise of enzymes along with fractionation of components of the total enzyme aid in the diagnosis. Figure 4.6 illustrates the patterns of enzyme rise after myocardial injury. *Creatine phosphokinase (CPK)* rises the earliest. A myocardial fraction, (MB [CK-MB]) can be detected and is highly specific for myocardial injury. Other conditions which may

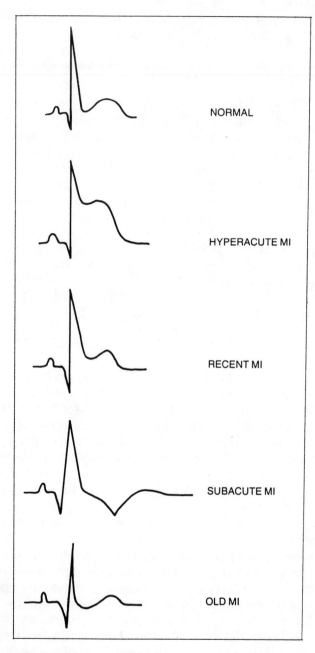

Figure 4.5.

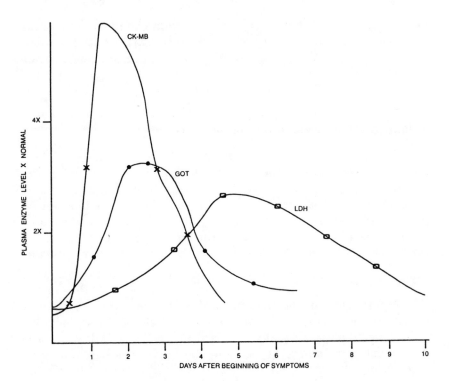

Figure 4.6.

cause a significant rise in CK–MB are associated with severe skeletal muscle injury of rhabdomyolysis, muscular dystrophy, dermatomyositis and hypothermia. *Lactic dehydrogenase (LDH)* is last to rise. It too may be fractionated into a myocardial fraction. Similar to LDH pattern elevations may occur with hemolysis, severe anemias, or renal disease.

Myocardial Scan

Myocardial scan with an agent known to be avid for injured myocardial cells is possible with Technetium-99M stannous pyrophosphate. In acute infarction the maximum myocardial uptake of Technetium-99M pyrophosphate by the myocardium occurs approximately 48 to 72 hours after onset of symptoms. If imaging is performed at the optimal time, a sensitivity of over 95% can be achieved for transmural infarction and somewhat less for nontransmural infarction. Cardiac imaging is most useful in evaluating patients in whom the diagnosis of infarction cannot otherwise be made, as with bundle branch block on the ECG, or after cardiac enzymes have already returned to normal, since the cardiac scan may remain positive for as long as two weeks after an acute infarction.

Treatment of Myocardial Infarction

The routine care of the acute MI includes hospitalization in a coronary care unit for the first 24-48 hours for monitoring and treatment of pain. Following the recovery from the acute phase, efforts towards rehabilitation should be instituted including slowly progressive ambulation, education concerning the nature of the disease and plans for evaluation concerning the extent of infarctin and the presence of other underlying coronary artery disease.

Complications

Major effort in the treatment of MI is directed towards identification and management of the complications. These include:
Arrhythmias: Virtually all persons with an MI will have *ventricular premature beats,* and these are most commonly successfully treated with intravenous lidocaine. Ventricular arrhythmias beyond the first 48 hours usually require long term oral anti-arrhythmic treatment. *Atrial premature beats* may occur and usually do not require treatment. Atrial flutter or fibrillation is managed with digitalis and quinidine or procainamide, if necessary. *Sinus bradycardia* usually occurs in the setting of an inferior wall myocardial infarction and, if hemodynamically significant, is managed with intravenous atropine. *Second and third degree heart block* may also occur. These are more benign if they occur in an inferior myocardial infarction and may not require treatment if there is an adequate ventricular response and no hemodynamic derangement. A temporary standby pacemaker placed in the right ventricle may be necessary. Usually the heart block reverses in less than a week.

Congestive Heart Failure may result from an MI if the damage is extensive. This is managed with diuretic, digitalis and sodium restriction.

Cardiogenic Shock is present if there is decreased systemic blood pressure (less than 90 mm Hg) and decreased peripheral perfusion. It is diagnosed with a pulmonary artery catheter (Swan-

Ganz catheter) showing a pulmonary wedge pressure above 20 mm Hg, cardiac index below 2.5 L/min/M2 and systolic arterial blood pressure below 90 mm Hg. It is treated with the intravenous inotropic agents dopamine or dobutamine. If this is unsuccessful, intraaortic balloon pump augmentation of arterial blood pressure and diastolic blood flow is warranted. The prognosis of cardiogenic shock is poor despite these measures.

Pericarditis which is inflammation of the sac lining the heart is recognized in approximately 20% of patients with MI. It is diagnosed by the presence of a friction rub over the precordium. It may result in chest pain and often requires analgesics. The presence of pericariditis is a contraindication to the continuation of anticoagulants which may cause a bloody pericardial effusion and possibly pericardial tamponade.

Dressler's Syndrome (postmyocardial infarction syndrome) is a febrile pleuropericarditis which may arise between 10 days to 2-3 months after an infarction. It is primarily characterized by chest pain which can usually be relieved by salicylates and, failing this, with opiates. It's thought to be an autoimmunophenomenon and be successfully treated with corticosteroids.

Ventricular Aneurysm which is a bulging area in the infarcted region may develop if the injury has been extensive. It will develop after several weeks and be associated with other complications such as peripheral embolization, ventricular arrhythmias and heart failure if the damage is extensive. Aneurysms usually do not rupture and in the absence of the above complications, require no specific treatment.

Papillary Muscle Infarction and Rupture may occur after an MI and result in severe mitral regurgitation and heart failure. Diagnosis is confirmed by cardiac catheterization with a flow directed (Swan-Ganz) catheter which shows a large "V" wave in the pulmonary wedge pressure tracing. If possible, surgical insertion of a prosthetic valve is delayed for 3 or more weeks to allow some healing of the infarcted myocardium.

Interventricular Septum Rupture may occur if there is extensive infarction of the septum. It is recognized by the presence of a new systolic murmur at the left sternal edge. If the perforation is low in the septum, the murmur may be loudest midway between the septum and cardiac apex and be confused with papillary muscle rupture. Heart catheterization will demonstrate an increase in oxygenation of right ventricular blood ("step-up" in oxygen saturation when compared to the right atrial blood).

Prognosis

Prognosis in myocardial infarction is frequently estimated by the following classification:

Class I: Myocardial infarction uncomplicated by clinical evidence of left ventricular failure.

Class II: Mild to moderate left ventricular failure as judged by either basilar rales, presence of an S-3 gallop, and/or a chest x-ray which shows evidence of pulmonary congestion.

Class III: Severe left ventricular failure as manifested by rales up to the apices of the chest, or lcinical and radiographic evidence of frank pulmonary edema.

Class IV: Cardiogenic shock as manifested by a systolic blood pressure of less than 90 mm Hg, associated with evidence of circulatory insufficiency.

Prevention

Preventing mortality and morbidity after myocardial infarction has been extensively studied over the past few years. Table 4.3 lists causes of death after MI and potential beneficial interventions.

SUDDEN CARDIAC DEATH (SCD)

Sudden cardiac death is the most common cause of death in those with coronary artery disease. It should be remembered, however, that coronary artery disease is not the only cause for sudden cardiac death. Table 4.4 lists causes of sudden cardiac death in the absence of coronary artery disease.

However, in the majority of patients who die of SCD there is extensive occlusive atherosclerotic disease of major epicardial coronary vessels. There are two sudden cardiac death syndromes. These are illustrated in Table 4.5.

The syndrome of acute myocardial infarction has already been covered earlier in this chapter. It appears to be precipitated by thrombotic occlusion or rupture of a coronary vessel plaque.

The syndrome of electrical failure presents as one of three electrical patterns:

1) Ventricular fibrillation
2) Ventricular tachycardia

TABLE 4.3
CAUSES OF DEATH AFTER MI
AND POTENTIAL INTERVENTIONS

Mechanism	Intervention
Progressive coronary atherosclerosis	Risk factor intervention
Coronary thrombosis	Anticoagulants
Recurrent ischemia	Nitrates Beta blockers Calcium channel blockers
Congestive heart failure	Inotropics Preload, afterload reduction
Ventricular fibrillation	Anti-arrhythmics

TABLE 4.4
CAUSES OF SUDDEN CARDIAC DEATH
IN THE ABSENCE OF CORONARY ARTERY DISEASE

I. CONGENITAL HEART DISEASE
  A. Structural abnormalities (hypoplastic left heart, VSD, etc.)
  B. Electrical abnormalities
    1. Sinotrial node disease
    2. Atrioventricular node disease
    3. Accessory bypass tracts with tachyarrhythmias
    4. Hereditary Q-T prolongation
      a. Jervell and Lange-Nielsen syndromes
      b. Romano-Ward syndrome

II. ACQUIRED HEART DISEASE
  A. Acute pericardial tamponade (trauma)
  B. Myocardial disease
    1. Cardiomyopathy
    2. Myocarditis
    3. Infiltrative disease (hemochromatosis, amyloid, etc.)
    4. Degeneration of conduction system (Lenegre's, Lev's)
    5. Metastatic malignant disease
    6. Cardiac tumors
  C. Valvular disease
    1. Bacterial endocarditis
    2. Mitral valve prolapse syndrome
    3. Aortic stenosis
    4. Prosthetic valve malfunction
  D. Coronary embolism
  E. Cardiac rupture (trauma)

TABLE 4.5
TWO SUDDEN CARDIAC DEATH SYNDROMES

Myocardial Infarction	*Electrical Failure*
Warning signs present	Absent
Thrombosis of coronary artery	Absent
ECG and enzyme changes of MI	Absent
Premature ventricular contractions	Present
Low recurrence of V-fib	High recurrence

3) Brachcardia-Asystole

The first two of these are more likely to be successfully treated (defibrillation for V-fib and anti-arrhythmics such as lidocaine for V-tach). The last, Bradycardia-Asystole appears to be the sign of a seriously impaired heart.

Patients who have previously been resuscitated from SCD are at a great risk of having a recurrent episode. Also, these patients frequently have a significant number of complex premature ventricular complexes (PVCs) as a premonitory sign of the risk of SCD. Consequently, several techniques have been developed to attempt to predict, on the basis of the presence of frequent complex PVCs, the risk of SCD. These techniques include:

Exercise stress testing to provoke PVCs (see chapter two).

Ambulatory (Holter) monitoring (see chapter two).

Electrophysiologic testing (EPS): This technique consists of passing a temporary pacemaker to the heart and programming extrasystoles to occur in an attempt to predict the vulnerability to the development of V-fib and V-tach. Figure 4.7 illustrates a pacing sequence during an EPS where ventricular tachycardia was elicited by a single programmed extrasystole. Once this vulnerability is demonstrated, various anti-arrhythmic drug regimens are instituted until the arrhythmia can no longer be elicited.

CONGESTIVE HEART FAILURE (CHF)

Coronary artery disease may present as congestive heart failure. The clinical features are essentially the same as those reviewed in chapter five, i.e., dyspnea, rales and gallops. Treatment of CHF in coronary artery disease is essentially the same, as CHF from other causes with precautions to be certain that the treatment does not impair the myocardial oxygen supply/demand ratio.

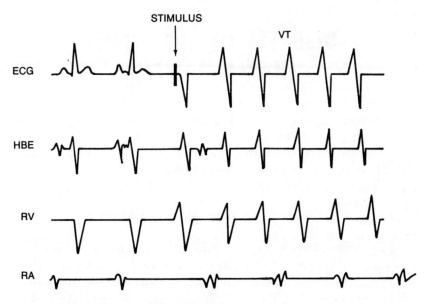

Figure 4.7. Abbreviation: VT = ventricular tachycardia.

Chapter 5

DISEASES OF THE PUMP
(Heart Muscle)

Diseases of the pump or heart muscle are termed "cardiomyopathy." There are three major categories of these diseases: 1) Congestive cardiomyopathy, 2) hypertrophic cardiomyopathy (IHSS), and 3) restrictive cardiomyopathy.

CONGESTIVE CARDIOMYOPATHY

The characteristic pathophysiologic abnormality in the congestive cardiomyopathies is a failure of systolic or pump function. Patients with this condition usually present with heart failure, arrhythmias, or peripheral emboli. The left ventricle, which is grossly dilated, contracts poorly, and there is a marked decrease in ejection fraction associated with increased end-systolic and end-diastolic volumes.

Table 5.1 lists some of the known causes of congestive cardiomyopathy.

Clinical and Hemodynamic Findings

Examination of the heart of a patient with congestive cardiomyopathy reveals left ventricular enlargement. There may also be right ventricular enlargement if there is heart failure. Heart murmurs of mitral regurgitation and tricuspid regurgitation may be present. The cardiac apical pulse may be very prominent with a quadruple or triple impulse resulting from overfilling. These pulses are the sensory counterpart of gallops. Auscultation reveals a persistent triple or quadruple rhythm resulting from S3 and S4 gallops. The ECG is usually abnormal and varies from minor nondiagnostic ST-T waves to left ventricular hypertrophy or bundle branch blocks. The chest x-ray will frequently reveal cardiac

70

TABLE 5.1.
CAUSES OF MYOCARDIAL DISEASE

I. IDIOPATHIC
   A. Familial
   B. Peripartal (postpartal)
   C. Endocardial fibroelastosis
   D. Endomyocardial fibrosis

II. SECONDARY CARDIOMYOPATHY
   A. Neuromuscular diseases
      1. Friedrich's ataxia
      2. Muscular dystrophy
   B. Connective tissue diseases
   C. Neoplastic heart disease (primary or metastatic)
   D. Metabolic diseases (thyrotoxicosis, myxedema, etc.)
   E. Infiltrative diseases (amyloid, hemochromotosis, sarcoid, etc.)
   F. Nutritional diseases (beriberi, kwashiokor)
   G. Myocarditis (viral, bacterial, protozoal, parasitic)
   H. Toxic (uremia, alcohol, cobalt, adriamycin, phenothiazines)

enlargement and increased pulmonary vascular markings consistent with congested lung fields.

The other diseases which may present with a similar clinical picture and which must be differentiated from congestive cardiomyopathy are: hypertensive heart disease, congestive heart failure from coronary artery disease, rheumatic heart disease and pericardial disease.

On cardiac catheterization the left ventricle is found to be dilated and flabby with poor systolic performance. This is illustrated in Figure 5.1. The echocardiogram is also very useful in making the diagnosis. In congestive cardiomyopathy, the entire left ventricle is found to be dilated and poorly contracting, and this finding helps to make the diagnosis, although coronary artery disease cannot be ruled out without coronary arteriography. Figure 5.2 illustrates an M-mode echo of a patient with congestive cardiomyopathy.

Treatment

Treatment of congestive cardiomyopathy is often difficult. If a specific cause is found, it must be specifically treated; however,

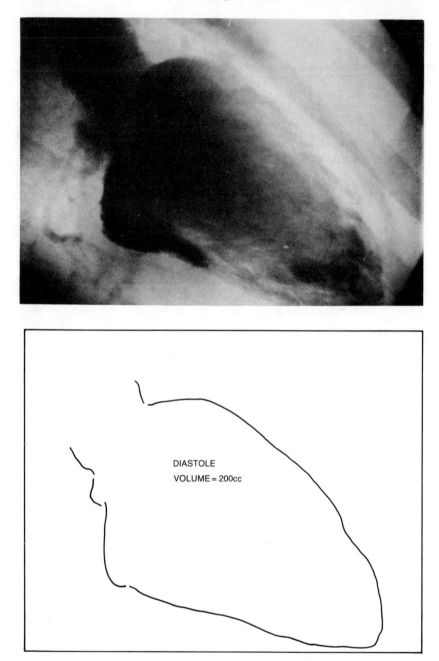

Figure 5.1A.

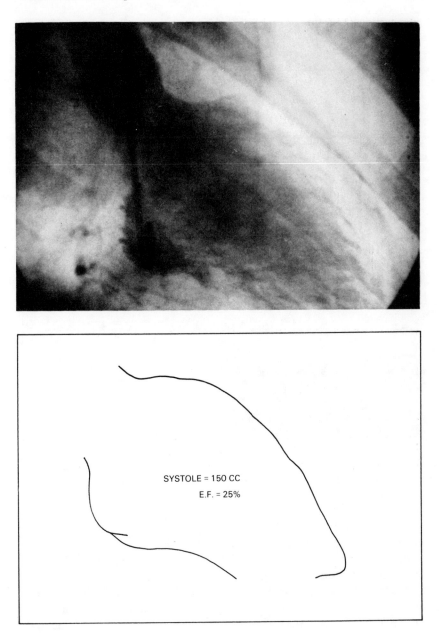

SYSTOLE = 150 CC

E.F. = 25%

Figure 5.1 B.

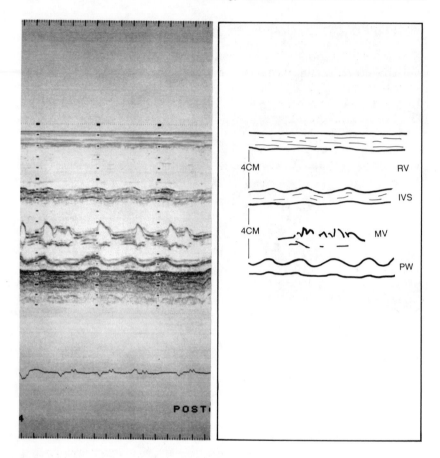

Figure 5.2. Abbreviations: RV = right ventricle; IVS = interventricular septum; MV = mitral valve; PW = posterior wall.

in most cases the patient will present with failure, and no specific etiologic agent is ever found. The manifestations of cardiomyopathy are treated with digitalis, diuretic, afterload reducing agents and appropriate anti-arrhythmics. Myocardial biopsy may detect on-going myocarditis and adrenal steroids and anti-metabolites are currently being tried. If peripheral embolization has occurred, anticoagulant therapy is warranted if not otherwise contraindicated. As a last resort, cardiac transplantation may be considered in the appropriate patient.

Prognosis

Prognosis in idiopathic congestive cardiomyopathy is difficult to predict. Approximately 3/4 of patients will have an accelerated course to death with 2/3 of the deaths occurring within the first 2 years after diagnosis. Approximately 20% of the patients will have clinical improvement.

HYPERTROPHIC (OBSTRUCTIVE) CARDIOMYOPATHY
(Idiopathic Hypertrophic Subaortic Stenosis [IHSS])

The characteristic pathologic feature of the hypertrophic cardiomyopathies is ventricular septal hypertrophy. The other walls of the ventricle may be normal, however the basal portion of the septum is hypertrophied to a degree where it may impede emptying of the ventricle during systole. The ejection fraction tends to be increased due to the occlusive effect of the septal hypertrophy, and the end–diastolic pressure is frequently elevated. Patients may have obstruction to outflow at rest or the obstruction may develop with provocation.

Figure 5.3 illustrates the pathologic picture of IHSS with the accompanying M–mode echo and Figure 5.4 the hemodynamic pattern of obstruction to flow within the ventricular cavity.

Clinical Picture

These patients present with dyspnea, angina pectoris, presyncope, syncope, palpitations or arrhythmias and more rarely, congestive heart failure. The heart failure usually occurs with the onset of atrial fibrillation because of the loss of atrial contraction and the shortened diastolic filling time resulting in marked elevation in pulmonary venous pressure with resultant pulmonary congestion.

A systolic murmur is usually present and is thought to result both from the obstruction to ventricular outflow and from mitral regurgitation. The mitral regurgitation results from the anterior mitral leaflet being pulled into the ventricular outflow tract during systole due to the Venturi effect of the increased velocity of blood across the area of the hypertrophied septum. The murmur is usually loudest in the second, third and fourth intercostal spaces to the left of the sternum or at the cardiac apex.

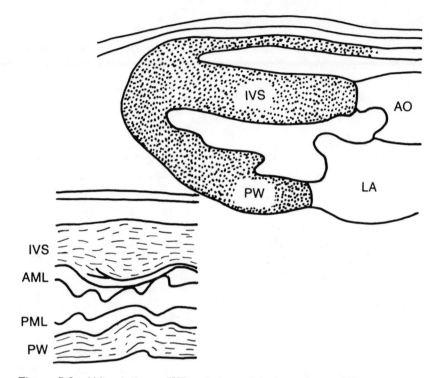

Figure 5.3. Abbreviations: IVS = interventricular septum; PW = posterior wall; AML = anterior mitral leaflet; PML = posterior mitral leaflet; LA = left atrium.

Any maneuver which decreases the size of the already narrowed ventricular outflow tract will increase the degree of obstruction and the loudness of the murmur. Consequently the following will increase the intensity of the murmur of IHSS: 1) valsalva, 2) standing, and 3) amyl nitrate.

If ventricular contractility is increased, the obstruction may also increase and the intensity of the murmur will increase. This may occur with infusion of isoproterenol (beta agonist) or digitalis.

Maneuvers which decrease the obstruction and the intensity of the murmur are squatting and peripheral vasoconstrictors (raises afterload).

Other clinical features of IHSS are:

1) Double carotid pulse, rising rapidly in early systole, then suddenly cutting off in midsystole and then rise to a lower level in late systole (Spike and Dome).

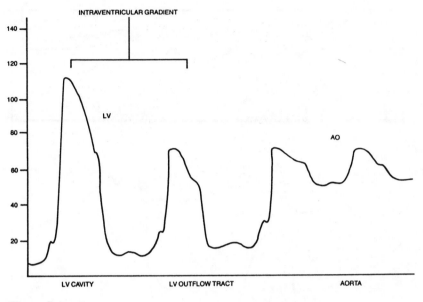

Figure 5.4.

    2)   Double apex pulse beat.
    3)   Loud S4 gallop.
Figure 5.5 illustrates these features.

    The M-mode echocardiogram shows a characteristic picture of: 1) Hypertrophied septum (assymmetric septal hypertrophy), and 2) systolic anterior motion of the anterior mitral leaflet (SAM) (Figure 5.3).

Treatment

    Treatment of IHSS consists of administration of B-adrenergic blocking agents or calcium channel antagonists (most commonly verapamil) in an effort to decrease the degree of outflow obstruction. It is generally agreed that digitalis should not be given to these patients unless there is heart failure or atrial fibrillation. The symptoms of the disease may be aggravated by the use of nitrates. Surgery has been successful in some cases where the degree of outflow obstruction is life-threatening or seriously symptomatic. Appropriate anti-arrhythmics are used for demonstrated arrhythmias.

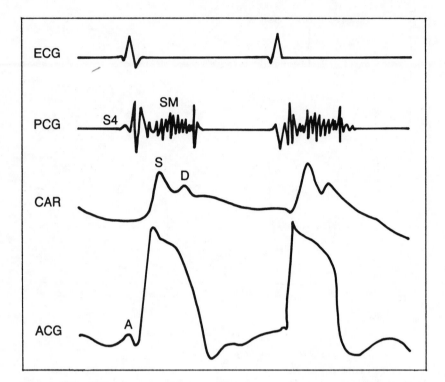

Figure 5.5. Abbreviations: PCG = phonocardiogram; CAR = carotid pulse tracing; ACG = apexcardiogram; S = spike; D = dome; SM = systolic murmur.

RESTRICTIVE CARDIOMYOPATHY

The hemodynamic pattern of restrictive cardiomyopathy is characterized by an elevated filling pressure in the ventricles associated with normal or nearly normal systolic function. This distinguishes it from congestive cardiomyopathy which has elevated filling pressures but poor systolic function. The restrictive process is due to infiltration of the myocardium from conditions such as: amyloidosis, sarcoidosis, hemochromatosis, Leoffler's eosinophilic endomyocardial disease and endomyocardial fibrosis. Except for hemochromatosis, these conditions have no known specific therapy and are associated with progressive deterioration and a grave prognosis.

Table 5.2 illustrates hemodynamic features which distinguish the three types of cardiomyopathy.

TABLE 5.2
LEFT VENTRICULAR FUNCTION
IN PRIMARY CARDIOMYOPATHIES

	Congestive	*Restrictive*	*Hypertrophic*
Volumes	Increased	Normal	Normal or Decreased
Ejection Fraction	Decreased	Normal	Normal or Increased
Wall Thickness	Normal or Increased	Normal	Increased
End-diastolic Pressure	Normal or Increased	Increased	Increased

Chapter 6

DISEASES OF THE VALVES

A useful approach to understanding valvular heart disease is to consider the disorders of the left and right INFLOW and OUT-FLOW tracts. There are essentially two major disorders of the inflow and outflow tracts: *stenosis* and *incompetence*. While incompetence occurs at the valvular level, stenosis may also occur below or above the valve. The most frequently seen clinical abnormalities of the left ventricular outflow tract are: *aortic stenosis, aortic incompetence,* and *muscular subvalvular stenosis* (IHSS — see chapter five). In the inflow tract, the most common lesions are *mitral stenosis, mitral regurgitation,* and *mitral valve prolapse.*

LEFT VENTRICULAR OUTFLOW TRACT

Aortic Stenosis (AS)

Etiology

The etiology of aortic stenosis may vary depending on the presence of other valvular involvement and age of the patient. Isolated aortic valve disease is rarely, if ever, rheumatic. The unicuspid valve is the most common cause of isolated aortic stenosis in children and in young adults, the bicuspid valve presents with stenosis usually at middle age and aortic sclerosis is the most common cause of isolated AS in elderly patients, particularly over age 65.

Symptoms

There is a classic triad of symptoms in severe aortic stenosis:
1) Effort syncope
2) Angina pectoris
3) Dyspnea (left ventricular failure)

The symptoms generally appear later in the course of the disease (e.g., when compared to mitral stenosis). Sudden death may occur with aortic stenosis without preceding symptoms in 3–5% of cases. This complication is, however, more likely to occur during the symptomatic stage of the disease (incidence is 15–20%). Shortness of breath due to left ventricular failure is the most serious symptom with death occurring within 1–3 years after the onset. Eighty percent mortality has been observed within 4 years of onset of any of these symptoms.

Physical Examination

A physical examination is very helpful. The pertinent findings are:

1) Pulsus parvus and tardus (decreased volume and upstroke of carotid pulse).

2) Thrill over the precordium may be palpable.

3) Ejection sound (loud in congenital AS, and soft in rheumatic AS).

4) Single or paradoxical splitting of S2.

5) S4 gallop.

A long systolic crescendo/decrescendo murmur which is most audible at the aortic area, left sternal edge or occasionally at the apex (see chapter three for diagram of ejection murmur). When the AS becomes severe, the murmur may peak late in systole. The murmur radiates to the carotid.

The systolic blood pressure is usually low, and the diastolic pressure is essentially normal (narrow pulse pressure).

Figure 6.1 illustrates the murmur, carotid pulse and apex recording of a patient with AS. The apex recording, which is merely a displacement recording from the apex of the left ventricle, reveals a large "a" wave indicating a stiff myocardium.

Laboratory Findings

The chest x-ray may show normal or increased size of the left ventricle. In the elderly there may be calcification of the aortic valve. There is frequently dilatation of the ascending aorta. Figure 6.2 shows a drawing depicting calcium in the region of the aortic valve on a lateral chest x-ray.

The ECG demonstrates left ventricular hypertrophy. Left bundle branch block, left atrial enlargement and left axis deviation may also be present.

The echocardiogram may show dilated aortic root and increased density of echoes of the aortic leaflets with decreased opening. Figure 6.3 illustrates an echo consistent with AS.

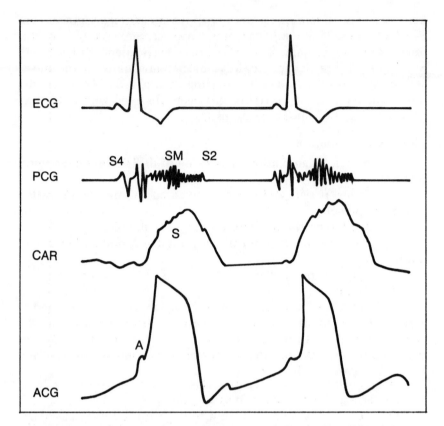

Figure 6.1. Abbreviations: SM = systolic murmur; S = shudder; PCG = phono-cardiogram; CAR = carotid pulse tracing; ACG = apexcardiogram; S = spike; D = dome; SM = systolic murmur.

Cardiac catheterization reveals a significant pressure drop (gradient) across the aortic valve. The aortic valvular area is calculated in severe AS to be less than 0.9 cm2 (normal valvular area is 3–4 cm2).

Treatment

Asymptomatic Patients: Such patients require bacterial endocarditis prophylaxis and instructions to avoid strenuous exertion.

Symptomatic Patients: Digoxin is usually the treatment of choice for congestive heart failure. Diuretics must be used care-

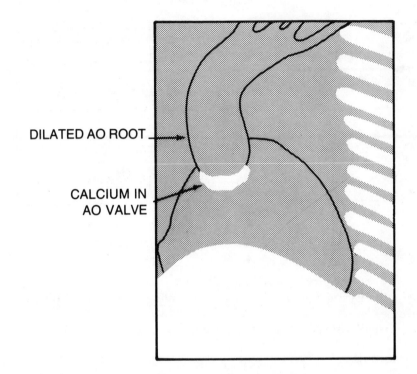

DILATED AO ROOT

CALCIUM IN
AO VALVE

Figure 6.2.

fully, because the heart with AS is relatively sensitive to preload, and marked diuresis may result in significant drop in cardiac output and result in hypotension. All symptomatic patients should have cardiac catheterization. Aortic valve replacement is recommended if the aortic valvular area is calculated to be less than 1 cm2. Arrhythmias are managed with appropriate anti-arrhythmics. Angina pectoris may be managed with nitrates.

Aortic Insufficiency (AI)

Etiology

The following are usual causes of aortic insufficiency:
1) Rheumatic endocarditis
2) Bacterial endocarditis
3) Collagen vascular disease, namely Reiter's disease and ankylosing spondylitis

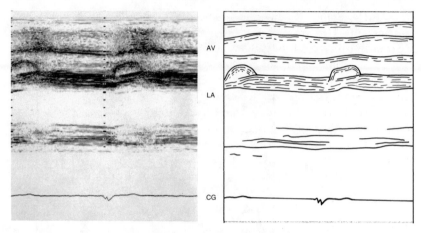

Figure 6.3. Abbreviations: AV = aortic valve; LA = left atrium.

4)   Congential bicuspid aortic valve
5)   Cystic medial necrosis of ascending aorta (Marfan's syndrome)
6)   Severe systemic hypertension

Symptoms

Symptoms of aortic insufficiency include:
1)   Angina pectoris (less common than in AS)
2)   Left ventricular failure (dyspnea, etc.)
The usual onset of symptoms in chronic aortic regurgitation is 10 or more years after diagnosis.

Physical Examination

The arterial pulse is very revealing in aortic incompetence. The hemodynamics are characterized by increased volume of blood ejected into the aorta during systole and increased distal runoff in diastole. This has resulted in the description of several types of pulses in aortic insufficiency.
Corrigan's Pulse: Abruptly rising and falling pulsation.
Demusset's Sign: Rhythmic nodding of the head synchronous with the heart beat.
Quincke's Sign: Alternate reddening and blanching of the nail bed with each heart beat.
Duroziez's Murmur: Biphasic bruit detectable in the femoral artery by applying moderate pressure with a stethoscope.

Hill's Sign: Exaggerated systolic pressure in the femoral arteries (60-100 mm Hg) more than that in the brachial arteries (normally up to 20 mm Hg).

Precordial palpation reveals enlargement of the left ventricle and prominently bounding and diffuse *left ventricular impulse* (due to increased volume of blood passing through the ventricle).

Auscultation discloses a characteristic high frequency early decrescendo diastolic murmur (see chapter three and Figure 6.4). The murmur's length correlates reasonably well with severity of regurgitation in chronic valvular disease. In addition a diastolic rumble (Austin Flint rumble) is frequently heard in significant aortic regurgitation. An S3 gallop is frequently present.

Laboratory Findings

The *ECG* usually shows left ventricular hypertrophy in significant AI.

The *chest x-ray* demonstrates left ventricular dilatation and dilatation of the ascending aorta (Figure 6.5).

The *echocardiogram* shows increased left ventricular volume, hyperdynamic motion of the ventricular walls and fluttering of the

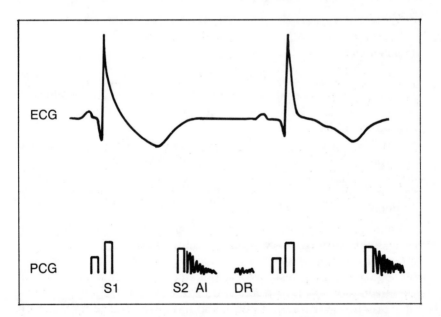

Figure 6.4. Abbreviations: AI = aortic insufficiency; DR = diastolic rumble.

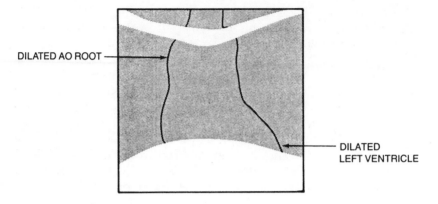

DILATED AO ROOT

DILATED
LEFT VENTRICLE

Figure 6.5.

mitral valve (Figure 6.6). In severe aortic incompetence, there may be premature closure of the mitral valve.

Cardiac catheterization demonstrates the regurgitation through the aortic valve during diastole, and the dilated left ventricle.

Management

Medical management includes bacterial endocarditis prophylaxis, anti-streptococcal prophylaxis in children or young adults if the AI is of rheumatic origin, digitalis and diuretics in patients with heart failure.

It is critical to operate and replace the aortic valve in aortic incompetence prior to the development of ventricular decompensation. This may be difficult to diagnose because of the long standing ventricular dilatation. Signs which may be helpful in making the decision to replace the valve are:

Early closure of the mitral valve on echocardiography because this indicates very severe incompetence.

Left ventricular systolic dimension more than 55 mm because this indicates failing systolic performance of the ventricle.

Decreased ejection fraction on exercise. Cardiac imaging indicates potential ventricular failure and has been used to indicate the need for valve replacement.

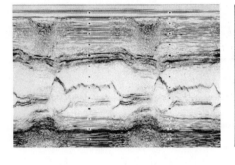 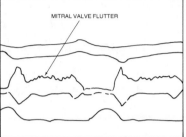

MITRAL VALVE FLUTTER

Figure 6.6.

LEFT VENTRICULAR INFLOW TRACT

Mitral Stenosis (MS)

Etiology

The rheumatic process is the most common cause of mitral stenosis. Less frequent causes are: congenital mitral stenosis, left atrial myxoma, viral infection of the valve, calcification of the mitral valvular annulus.

Hemodynamic Changes in Mitral Stenosis

The left ventricular end–diastolic pressure is normal or low due to inadequate filling during diastole. The pressure drop (gradient) across the mitral valve is usually between 5-30 mm Hg depending on the severity of the stenosis and flow across the valve. The left atrium is enlarged when the stenosis is severe and pulmonary artery pressure is frequently elevated (pulmonary hypertension).

Symptoms

1) Paroxysmal nocturnal dyspnea
2) Dyspnea on exertion
3) Hemoptysis
4) Chest pain (resembling angina or pleuritic pain)
5) Palpitations (due to atrial fibrillation)

Physical Examination

Pertinent findings upon physical examination are:
1) Diastolic rumbling murmur
2) Opening snap of mitral valve
3) Accentuated first heart sound
4) Accentuated P-2 if pulmonary hypertension is present
Figure 6.7 illustrates the auscultatory complex of MS.

Laboratory Findings

The *ECG* will show left atrial enlargement ("p mitrale"), evidence of right ventricular hypertrophy (if pulmonary hypertension is present), and, perhaps later in the course, atrial fibrillation.

The *chest x-ray* will show left atrial enlargement (characterized by straightened or bulging heart border below the silhouette of the left pulmonary artery, double density behind the right atrium and elevated left mainstem bronchus). There may also be calcification of the mitral valve, enlargement of the left and right main pulmonary arteries, and evidence for interstitial edema.

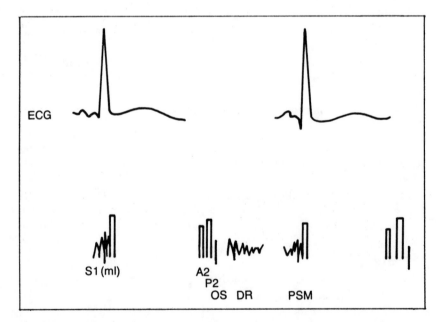

Figure 6.7. Abbreviations: OS = opening snap; DR = diastolic rumble; PSM = presystolic murmur.

The *echocardiogram* is frequently very helpful in MS. It will show decreased closing slope of the mitral valve, thickening and perhaps calcification of the mitral valve (Figure 6.8). It will also show: decreased closing slope of the anterior mitral leaflet in diastole (E-F slope); inappropriate anterior motion of the posterior leaflet during diastole; thickened leaflets with decreased excursion; and dilated left atrium.

Cardiac catheterization in MS shows a transvalvular gradient. Mitral valve area (MVA) may be calculated, the normal area being 4-6 cm2.

$$\text{Mild MS} = \text{MVA of} \rangle = 1.5 \text{ cm2}$$
$$\text{Moderate MS} = \text{MVA of } 1 - 1.5 \text{ cm2}$$
$$\text{Severe stenosis} = \text{MVA of} \langle 1.0 \text{ cm2}$$

Management

Children and young adults with rheumatic heart disease should receive penicillin prophylaxis for beta hemolytic streptococcal infections. All patients should receive bacterial endocarditis prior to all dental and surgical procedures.

Atrial fibrillation is usually managed using digoxin and quinidine. Elective cardioversion is usually unsuccessful because of the enlarged atrium.

Surgery is indicated if the MVA is less than 1.0 cm2 or if there is symptomatic moderate stenosis. Possible surgical proce-

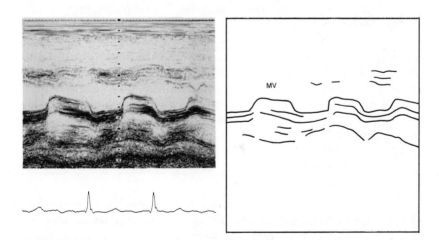

Figure 6.8. Abbreviation: MV = mitral valve.

dures include: mitral commissurotomy or mitral valve replacement with a prosthesis.

Natural History: An asymptomatic period of 10-20 years is usual following an attack of rheumatic fever. It takes only 5-10 years for most patients to progress from mild to total disabiltiy.

Mitral Regurgitation (MR)

Etiology

There are numerous causes of mitral regurgitation including:

Rheumatic — the leaflets are thickened and distorted causing incompetence of the valve.

Calcification of the annulus — occurs in the elderly population.

Bacterial endocarditis — destroys the valve structure.

Marfan's syndrome — myxomatous degeneration of the valve.

Ischemic — rupture of the papillary head or necrosis of the papillary muscle.

Left atrial myxoma — impairs the closing mechanism of the valve.

Congenital mitral regurgitation.

Mitral valve prolapse.

Pathophysiology

In patients with mitral regurgitation, the regurgitant volume is ejected into the left atrium prior to the opening of the aortic valve. The amount of regurgitation is partially determined by aortic pressure and is, therefore, greater in hypertensive patients, and smaller in patients with low systemic pressure. A large volume of mitral regurgitation produces only a minimum increase in myocardial oxygen consumption, consequently this lesion may be well tolerated for many years because the left ventricle operates at the high point of the Starling's curve, and the afterload is lower (the blood is ejected into both the aorta and the left atrium).

Symptoms

The symptoms do not usually develop in patients with chronic mitral regurgitation until the left ventricle fails. The time interval between the attack of rheumatic fever and the development of symptoms tends to be longer than mitral stenosis. In severe mitral regurgitation, the left atrial and pulmonary pressures are elevated causing:

1) Paroxysmal nocturnal dyspnea
2) Dyspnea on exertion
3) Nonspecific chest pain
4) Hemoptysis may rarely be present

In chronic mitral regurgitation fatigue and exhaustion (due to low cardiac output) are frequent complaints.

Physical Examination

Pulse volume may be decreased because blood is regurgitating backwards. Lungs may have rales of congestive heart failure. Apical impulse is brisk, diffuse and bouncing (due to the large left ventricular volume). This is usually the most important physical finding in evaluating the severity of mitral regurgitation. S2 may be widely split due to shortening of left ventricular ejection time. P2 may be accentuated if there is pulmonary hypertension. An S3 gallop is common due to the high volume flow.

The systolic murmur is classically holosystolic, commencing immediately follwoing S1. The murmur frequently radiates towards the axilla. See chapter three for a diagram of the systolic murmur of mitral insufficiency.

Figure 6.9 illustrates the auscultatory complex of mitral regurgitation.

Laboratory Findings

On *ECG* there is left atrial enlargement, and left ventricular hypertrophy. There may also be atrial fibrillation, and, if pulmonary hypertension is present, right ventricular hypertrophy.

On *chest x-ray* one sees cardiomegaly with left ventricular hypertrophy and left atrial enlargement. There may also be evidence for congestive heart failure in the lung fields with interstitial edema.

An important finding on the chest x-ray is *calcification of the mitral annulus* which gives away the etiology of the murmur (see Figure 6.10).

On *echocardiography* one finds enlarged left atrium and left ventricle which are not specific for mitral regurgitation. Findings which provide specific information concerning the underlying etiology include flail mitral leaflet and calcification of the mitral annulus (Figure 6.11).

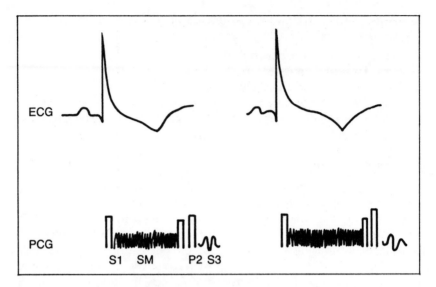

Figure 6.9. Abbreviation: SM = systolic murmur.

Management

Of all the usual measures employed in management of congestive heart failure, digitalis is much more important in MR than in mitral stenosis because of the volume overload. As usual diuretics are used for volume overload. Systolic unloading agents, as discussed in chapter four, may be employed if there is inadequate response to the above measures.

Surgical replacement of the mitral valve may be warranted if the volume overload of the heart has resulted in impairment of systolic function. The point in time at which this occurs is often difficult to determine. If surgery of a seriously incompetent valve is delayed too long, the left ventricle may be irreversibly damaged. Currently, serial echocardiograms are frequently employed to assess ventricular systolic performance and recommend surgical intervention when there is progressive enlargement in ventricular volume and decrease in systolic performance.

The *natural history* of mitral regurgitation depends upon the degree of damage to the valve and the consequent volume of regurgitation. The regurgitation may be well tolerated for many years. In one study, 80% of patients survived 5 years after diagnosis and 60% lived 10 years. If there is combined mitral stenosis, the prognosis is poorer.

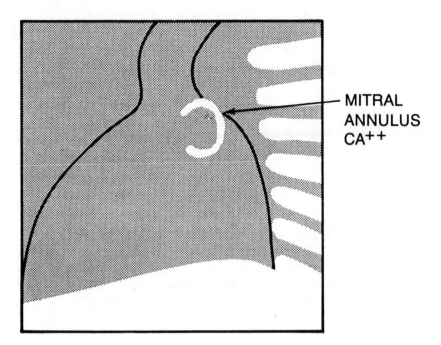

MITRAL
ANNULUS
CA^{++}

Figure 6.10.

Mitral Valve Prolapse (MVP)

Etiology

Mitral valve prolapse (Barlow's syndrome, Click–murmur syndrome) is a complex syndrome. The cardinal feature of this syndrome is a disproportion between the size of the left ventricular cavity and the length of the chordae tendineae. The function of chordae tendineae is to hold the mitral valvular leaflets in a proper position so that the valve is competent during systole. If the chordae tendineae are relatively long, the leaflets will prolapse into the atrium causing a click when their motion is checked. Frequently the leaflets become incompetent and a late systolic murmur is heard following the click. The full–blown picture of MVP appears to be caused by myxomatous degeneration of the valve, in which the spongiosa component of the valve proliferates and the quantity of acid mucopolysaccharide is increased.

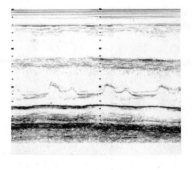 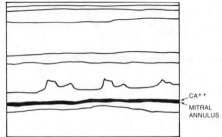

Figure 6.11.

Symptoms

The majority of patients are asymptomatic, however some patients complain of chest pain, which is atypical for angina pectoris, and palpitations.

The mechanical effects of the prolapsed valve leaflet striking the atrial wall during systole, or high tension on the papillary muscles or chordae tendineae, or mitral apparatus have been reasoned to be responsible for these symptoms.

Physical Examination

MVP has been found to be associated with other physical findings. Among them are: 1) narrow anterior–posterior diameter of the chest; pectus excavatum of the chest; and straight-back syndrome.

The characteristic findings on *cardiac auscultation* are mid-systolic click and late systolic murmur.

Any maneuver which decreases left ventricular volume, e.g., standing upright, valsalva maneuver, or amyl nitrate, will result in increased laxity of the valve apparatus and bring the click and murmur earlier in systole.

Laboratory Findings

On *ECG* there is frequently nonspecific ST–T wave changes. Also, there are often premature atrial and ventricular contractions. Paroxysmal tachycardias, supraventricular as well as ventricular, may also occasionally be found.

The *echocardiogram* is often very helpful in the diagnosis, revealing the late systolic buckling of the mitral valve (see Figure 6.12).

Cardiac catheterization is usually normal unless there is serious valve incompetence. On left ventricular angiography, the prolapse of the mitral valve may be demonstrated.

Treatment

Most patients with MVP have no significant symptoms and require no treatment, however several complications of the valve dysfunction have been described and should be managed. These include:

1) Significant arrhythmias — may require anti-arrhythmic treatment.

2) Significant chest pain — may respond to beta blockers. Occasionally a patient will have chest pain which is relieved by nitrates, although logically these agents should increase the degree of prolapse.

3) Transient ischemia attacks — have been associated with MVP and thought perhaps to be due to platelet thrombi. It is, therefore, recommended that these patients take anti-platelet agents (e.g., aspirin).

4) Bacterial endocarditis — has been found to occur in some patients with MVP. For this reason antibiotic bacterial endocarditis prophylaxis is warranted at the time of dental work or surgical procedures.

RIGHT VENTRICULAR OUTFLOW TRACT

Pulmonic Stenosis (PS)

Pulmonic stenosis is the most important disorder of the right ventricular outflow tract. It is usually congenital; however, in certain areas of the world (Mexico City), there is a high incidence of PS with rheumatic fever.

Symptoms

Most adult patients with mild to moderate PS (right ventricular systolic pressure between 75 and 100 mm Hg) are asymptomatic. If the pressure is more elevated than this, the symptoms of dyspnea, fatigue and chest pain may be present.

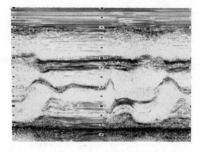 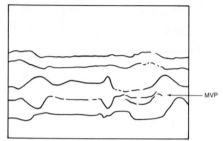

Figure 6.12. Abbreviation: MVP = mitral valve prolapse.

Physical Examination

On examination of the chest wall there is bulging and sustained right ventricular impulse along the left sternal edge. On auscultation there is characteristically a systolic *ejection sound* at the upper left sternal edge. P2 is diminished in intensity. A harsh diamond–shaped systolic ejection murmur, best heard at the upper left sternal border is present (see Figure 6.13).

Laboratory Findings

The *ECG* is frequently normal in mild cases. The presence of right ventricular hypertrophy indicates severe PS.

The *chest x–ray* shows evidence of right ventricular enlargement with post–stenotic dilatation of the main and left pulmonary arteries and decreased pulmonary vasculature.

On *echocardiogram* there will be enlargement of the right ventricle and increased a–wave of the pulmonic valve echo.

On *cardiac catheterization* a pressure drop (gradient) across the pulmonic valve is demonstrated.

Management

Asymptomatic patients with a right ventricular systolic pressure of 75 mm Hg or less are not candidates for surgery. Symptomatic patients with higher right ventricular systolic pressure are candidates of pulmonic valvuloplasty.

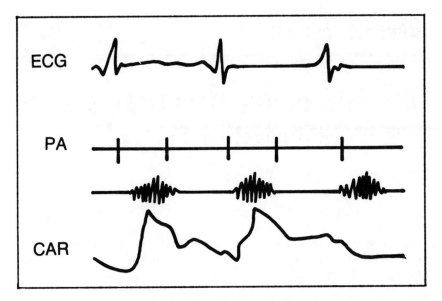

Figure 6.13. Abbreviations: PA = pulmonary area; CAR = carotid.

REFERENCES

1. Rapaport E: Natural history of aortic and mitral valve disease. *Am J Cardiol, 35:*221–227, 1975.

2. Spagnuolo M, Kloth H, Taranta A, Doyle E, Pasternack B: Natural history of rheumatic aortic regurgitations: Criteria predictive of death, congestive heart failure, and angina in young patients. *Circulation 44:*368–380, 1971.

3. Kirlin JW, Pacifico AD: Surgery for acquired valvular heart disease. *New Engl J Med, 288:*133–140, 1973.

4. Jeresaty RM: *Mitral Valve Prolapse.* New York: Raven Press, 1979.

5. Braunwald E: *Heart Disease: A Textbook of Cardiovascular Medicine.* Philadelphia: W.B. Saunders, 1980.

Chapter 7

DISEASES OF THE ELECTRICAL SYSTEM
(Conduction System)

ANATOMY AND PHYSIOLOGY

The anatomy and physiology of the conduction system was discussed in chapter one. It consists of the *major pacemaker*, the *sinoatrial node (SA node)*, the *atrioventricular node (AV node)*, the *bundle of His*, the *bundle branches* and the *terminal Purkinje fibers* (see Figure 7.1).

TACHYARRHYTHMIAS

There are many different classifications of tachyarrhythmias and this extensive list assails the student or physician when he or

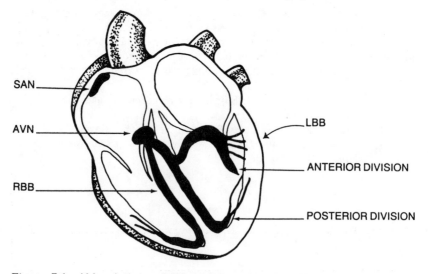

Figure 7.1. Abbreviations: SAN = sinoatrial node; AVN = atrioventricular node; RBB = right bundle branch; LBB = left bundle branch.

she is trying to make a specific diagnosis of an arrhythmia prior to instituting therapy. There are so many classifications and terms for the various tachyarrhythmias that the issue is frequently confused and inappropriate therapeutic choices are made.

Appropriate Therapy

In clinical practice in the treatment of acute arrhythmia, it is frequently not necessary to identify the specific site of the arrhythmia in order to choose appropriate therapy. This is because therapeutic choices are of a limited number, so one need only to determine two features of the arrhythmia prior to choosing the appropriate therapy. These features are the *manner of onset* of the arrhythmia, and whether the surface ECG has a *narrow or wide QRS* morphology.

Manner of Onset

One of the most important features of a tachyarrhythmia detected by continuous monitoring is the manner of onset. This will give a clue to the etiology of the arrhythmia and thus suggest appropriate treatment.

There are two accepted mechanisms of clinical arrhythmias: *increased automaticity* and *reentry*.

Increased Automaticity: Automaticity is the intrinsic ability of the specialized conduction system of the heart to undergo spontaneous phase 4 depolarization (Figure 7.2). These automatic cells

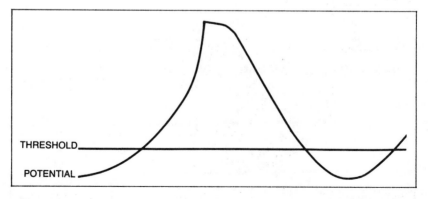

Figure 7.2.

spontaneously reach threshold potential then depolarize, recover, then the cycle repeats itself. The normal myocardium does not manifest spontaneous automaticity but will assume this characteristic if injured (1). The important feature of automaticity which allows classification is its manner of onset. It *slowly warms up* and progressively increases its firing rate until a new steady state is achieved. This is because automaticity is a normal feature of the specialized conducting system of the heart, and its increased firing rate is due to *external influences* such as hypoxia, hypokalemia, catecholamines, drugs (digitalis, theophylline, atropine) (1). Table 7.1 lists conditions and drugs which increase the firing rate of automatic cells.

A simple example of an automatic arrhythmia is sinus tachycardia associated with exercise. The sinus rate slowly and progressively increases during the exercise under the external influence of hypoxia and catecholamines and the balance of the sympathetic and parasympathetic nervous systems. A new steady state will be reached if the exercise is steady; then when the exercise is discontinued, the sinus rate will slowly return to normal.

Other automatic arrhythmias are: automatic atrial tachycardia, accelerated junctional rhythm, and accelerated ventricular rhythm.

Reentry: Reentrant arrhythmias, on the other hand, require a complex set of pathologic conditions before initiation. These are: 1) *dual pathways;* 2) *unidirectional block* in one of the pathways; and 3) *decremental conduction* in the other.

Figure 7.3 diagrams these features (2). In order for reentry to occur, block must occur in one pathway in one direction, and the

---

TABLE 7.1
CONDITIONS AND DRUGS WHICH ENHANCE AUTOMATICITY

Cathecholamines
Elevated extracellular calcium
Elevated extracellular potassium
Digitalis
Local ischemia
Hypoxia
Atropine
Theophylline

conduction in the other pathway must persist in order for the arrhythmia to be maintained.

Reentrant arrhythmias are usually initiated with a premature stimulus which finds one of the pathways totally refractory for antegrade conduction and then conducts slowly down the second pathway initiating the reentrant cycle. This is the manner in which programmed extrastimulation is used in the clinical electrophysiology laboratory to induce paroxysmal arrhythmias.

The major feature of the initiation of reentrant arrhythmia is the *abrupt onset,* starting with the premature systole. Either the

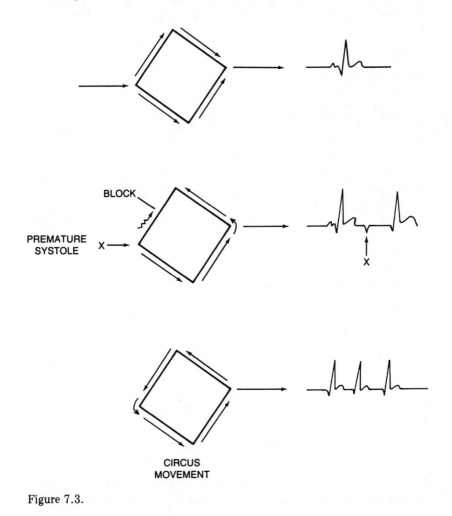

Figure 7.3.

patient's history or continuous monitoring may demonstrate the sudden change from a slow regular rhythm to a rapid rhythm without a warmup. This is the major distinguishing feature of reentry in contrast to an automatic arrhythmia.

Gradual onset — automatic arrhythmia.

Abrupt onset — reentrant arrhythmia.

Surface QRS Morphology

If the surface QRS morphology is narrow (less than 0.12 sec) then the tachyarrhythmia is originating above the AV junction which permits a normal sequence of conduction down the His-Purkinje system.

If the surface morphology is wide (more than 0.12 sec) then there are two possibilities: 1) the tachyarrhythmia originates below the AV junction, and the conduction throughout the ventricle takes an abnormal pathway. This arrhythmia is, of course, *ventricular tachycardia (VT)*. 2) The second possibility with a wide QRS tachyarrhythmia is the condition where the arrhythmia originates above the AV junction, but conduction through the His-Purkinje system is aberrant either because the rate is so fast that the impulse arrives during the refractory period of the bundle branch (usually the right bundle, though not invariably so), or secondly, because of pre-existing bundle branch block (Figure 7.4).

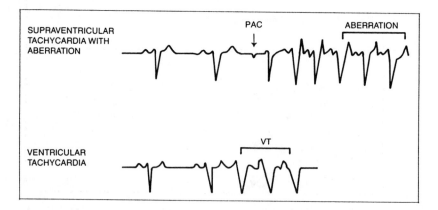

Figure 7.4. Abbreviations: PAC = premature atrial contraction; VT = ventricular tachycardia.

So, a wide QRS arrhythmia may be 1) ventricular tachycardia, or 2) supraventricular tachycardia with aberration or pre-existing bundle branch block.

We then arrive at a simple classification of tachyarrhythmias, illustrated in Figure 7.5.

Treatment

This simplified form of classification also simplifies treatment. All of the tacharrhythmias in Categories I and II are automatic arrhythmias and are usually driven by an external influence (see Table 7.1). No specific treatment of the arrhythmia is necessary until this external influence is identified and corrected. Automatic ventricular tachycardia is a pathologic arrhythmia and may result in symptoms of dizziness, if atrial contribution to systole is necessary to maintain cardiac output, however, the major therapeutic efforts should be directed at the external exciting influence.

Surface QRS

	Narrow	Wide
Gradual	I Sinus Tachy. Automatic atrial tachy. Accelerated junctional tachy	II All of I plus: Accelerated ventricular rhythm
Sudden	III PSVT: SA Node reentry Atrial reentry AV junctional reentry Reentry via bypass tract (WPW, LGL) Atrial flutter	IV All of III plus: Ventricular tachy.

(Left margin label: Manner of Onset)

Figure 7.5. Abbreviations: PSVT = paroxysmal supraventricular tachycardia; SA = sinoatrial; AV = atrioventricular; WPW = Wolff-Parkinson-White; LGL = Lown-Ganong-Levine.

Consequently the major clinical tachyarrhythmias will fall into Categories III and IV.

The first treatment of choice for all the arrhythmias in Category III is *verapamil*, the calcium channel antagonist. The reentry pathway in the majority of PSVTs involves the AV junction as a limb of the reentry circuit and verapamil will frequently prolong conduction through this portion of the loop enough to break the arrhythmia. Even if the AV junction is not a limb of the reentrant pathway, the rapid impulses pass through the junction to drive the ventricle, so an agent, such as verapamil, which slows conduction through this pathway will slow the ventricular response to the arrhythmia. Other agents which may break or control these arrhythmias are digitalis, B-blockers, procainamide, quinidine, disopyramide, and amiodarone.

A concern with this approach is that the occasional patient may have an increased ventricular rate after IV verapamil if the drug shortens the refractory period of the accessory pathway in preexcitation (see discussion later in this chapter). This is an unusual problem but possible. Some authors consider IV verapamil contraindicated in patients with atrial fibrillation just as digitalis may be contraindicated in the same situation (4).

Category IV includes all of the group III arrhythmias plus ventricular tachycardia (VT). Many publications have attempted to use surface morphology of the QRS to separate VT from PSVT with aberration. The best criteria are listed in Table 7.2. The feature which is the most helpful is atrioventricular dissociation, the demonstration that the atria and ventricles are beating independently.

If the patient has other evidence of organic heart disease, especially coronary artery disease or cardiomyopathy, then VT is statistically more probable than SVT.

The drug of choice in VT is lidocaine which has little effect on PSVT. The drug of second choice is procainamide followed by quinidine, disopramide, bretylium and possibly amiodarone.

If the arrhythmia is irregular, there are two other possibilities. These are:

1) *Atrial fibrillation*, which for practical purposes can be treated as a reentrant arrhythmia, although the mechanism is open to question; and

2) *Multifocal atrial tachycardia* which is an automatic rhythm in an abnormal atrial mileau and occurs commonly in

TABLE 7.2.
ECG FINDINGS HELPFUL IN DIFFERENTIATING SVT
WITH ABERRANT CONDUCTION FROM VT

WIDE QRS TACHYCARDIA

Suggests VT	*Suggests SVT with Aberration*
A-V dissociation	
Left axis deviation	
QRS width more than 0.14 sec	
If QRS of RBBB pattern:	
	Frontal plane axis between -30 and +120 degrees
Lead V-1: monophasic or biphasic QRS	Triphasic QRS
Lead V-6: R/S ratio less than 1	Initial negativity (q wave) followed by R wave with larger amplitude than S wave
If QRS of LBBB pattern:	
	Frontal plane axis between -30 and +90 degrees
Lead V-1: Initial R during tachycardia higher than initial R in sinus rhythm	Initial R during tachycardia lower than initial R during sinus rhythm
Lead V-6: qR complexes	

Reference (3)

respiratory failure. It can, for practical purposes, be treated as an automatic arrhythmia.

So, a simplified scheme of diagnosis and treatment is illustrated in Figure 7.6.

BRADYCARDIAS AND BLOCKS

Sick Sinus Syndrome (SSS)

Sick sinus syndrome (SSS) is a diagnosis often made when sinus bradycardia results from disease of the SA node. There may also be sinus arrest, sinoatrial block (block of the conduction of the impulses from the SA node), and, if the conduction system disease is more extensive, tachycardias and slow junctional escape

1) Slow onset + narrow or wide QRS → Look for external influences.

2) Abrupt onset + narrow QRS → Verapamil (5-10 mg IV)

3) Abrupt onset + wide QRS → Lidocaine (50-100 mg IV).

if fails:
  Procainamide
  or
  Verapamil may be tried as a therapeutic trial if PSVT is probable
  or
  Quinidine
  Disopyramide
  Bretylium
  Amiodarone

Figure 7.6.

rhythms. A variant of the sick sinus syndrome is atrial fibrillation with a slow ventricular response, because this is evidence of extensive conduction system disease involving the SA node, atria and AV node.

The symptoms of SSS include syncope, dizziness, fatigue, heart failure and evidence of poor peripheral perfusion (confusion, neurologic defects, renal dysfunction, etc.).

This diagnosis of SSS is made from the surface ECG finding of one of the above electrical disturbances (Figure 7.7) in a symptomatic patient. Occasionally the syndrome is intermittant and intracardiac pacing and recording is necessary to bring out the disturbances. Sinoatrial recovery time (SART) after pacing the atria may demonstrate long pauses (overdrive suppression) (Figure 7.8) of the sinoatrial node. Drugs such as atropine or isoproteronol may uncover such SA node abnormalities.

Treatment

The treatment of SSS consists of implantation of a demand pacemaker. Whether the pacemaker is an atrial or ventricular demand or atrio-ventricular sequential pacemaker is dependent upon the nature of the electrical disturbances and integrity of the AV node conduction.

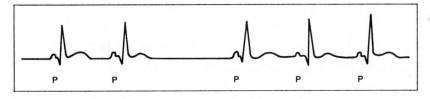

Figure 7.7.

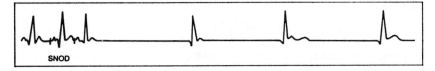

Figure 7.8. Abbreviation: SNOD = sinus node overdrive.

Atrioventricular Block

Block in the atrioventricular junction is of three types:
First degree: Prolonged PR interval
Second degree: Intermittant block
Third degree: Complete block

First Degree Block

First degree block (prolonged PR interval) (Figure 7.9) is asymptomatic and may be found in patients on digitalis or after an acute inferior wall myocardial infarction. The conduction time through the AV node is a function of three factors: 1) Inherent AV node refractoriness and conduction, 2) vagal (parasympathetic) stimulation which prolongs refractoriness and conduction, and 3) sympathetic stimulation which shortens refractoriness and conduction.

A prolonged PR interval at rest may often be simply converted to normal by standing or walking, because the increased sympathetic drive will then increase conduction rate.

Second Degree Block

Second degree block is divided into two types:
Mobitz I (Wenckebach) consisting of gradual progressive slowing of conduction until there is block. The conduction tissue

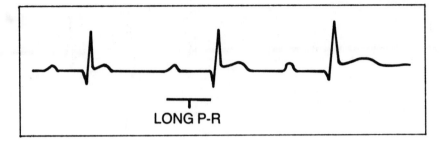

LONG P-R

Figure 7.9.

appears to fatigue, then give out. This is manifest on the ECG as cyclic gradual lengthening of the PR interval with shortening of the PR interval followed by a non-conducted p-wave (absent QRS) (Figure 7.10). Mobitz I is rarely associated with symptoms and is not an indication for a pacemaker.

Mobitz II consists of cyclic non-conducted p-waves *not* preceded by gradual lengthening of the PR interval. The PR interval may be normal or prolonged (Figure 7.11). Mobitz II indicates serious conduction system disease and is commonly associated with dizziness or syncope. It is an indication for permanent pacing because of the high incidence of subsequent complete heart block.

Third Degree Block

Third degree heart block consists of AV dissociation where p-waves are independent of QRS complexes (Figure 7.12). The QRS rate is usually slow, less than 50 bpm. If the block is low in the conduction system then the ventricle will be driven by a ventricular escape pacemaker with a wide QRS complex. If the block is high, the escape rhythm might come from the conduction tissue near the AV node and result in a narrow QRS. This escape rhythm may respond to vagal and sympathetic stimulation, and the patient may be asymptomatic. This type of complete AV block occurs as a congenital defect and may go unrecognized several years. It most commonly arises in children of mothers with connective tissue disease, e.g., systemic lupus erythematosis.

Third degree heart block is an indication for permanent cardiac pacing.

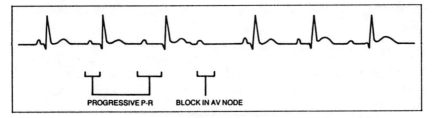

Figure 7.10.

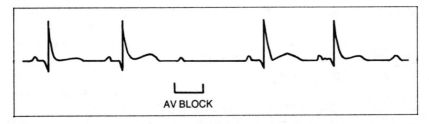

Figure 7.11.

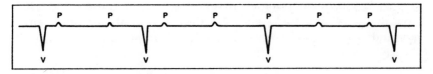

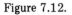

Figure 7.12.

Bundle Branch Blocks

Failure of impulse transmission either by the right or left bundle or by a major division of the left bundle may be expected to alter the sequence of activation of the ventricular mass and this changes the form and duration of the QRS complex. Figure 7.1 illustrates the major bundle branches and their divisions. The essential electrocardiographic elements in the definition of bundle branch block are:

1) Each QRS complex must be preceded regularly by a p-wave with a PR interval of 0.12 sec or more. (This criterion distinguishes bundle branch block from ectopic ventricular beats.)

2) QRS duration must be 0.12 sec or more.

3) In right bundle branch block there must be a tall late R

or R' wave in V–1 and a broad late S wave in I, V–5 and V–6 (Figure 7.13A).

In left bundle branch block there is an absent Q wave and a wide slurred or notched R wave in I, V–5 and V–6 (Figure 7.13B).

Right bundle branch block (RBBB) does not necessarily indicate other significant underlying cardiovascular disease and may be found in otherwise healthy persons.

Left bundle branch block (LBBB) is nearly always associated with organic heart disease including: coronary artery disease, hypertensive heart disease, aortic valve disease, cardiomyopathy, Lenegre's disease, Lev's disease or trauma.

There are usually no significant physiologic effects of the bundle branch blocks, however, LBBB may result in decreased ventricular contractility and cardiac output.

The intraventricular system is generally considered to be a trifascicular system, because the left bundle divides into the anterior and posterior divisions. Blocks of these individual divisions are known as *hemiblocks* or *fascicular blocks.*

Left Anterior Hemiblock

Left anterior hemiblock is suggested by the presence of QRS frontal plane axis between –30 deg. and –90 deg. inferiorly oriented initial QRS forces and QRS duration normal or only slightly prolonged.

Left Posterior Hemiblock

Left posterior hemiblock is suggested by the presence of QRS frontal plane axis between +80 deg. and +120 deg. and terminal forces are rightwardly directed. The same ECG pattern may be seen in right ventricular hypertrophy, pulmonary disease or vertical anatomic position of the heart, and these must be excluded prior to the diagnosis.

Trifascicular Disease

Trifascicular disease may be a harbinger of complete heart block and an indication for permanent pacing. Examples of trifascicular disease include:

1) RBBB + LAH + slowed conduction through the left posterior fascicle.

2) RBB + LPH + slowed conduction through the left anterior fascicle.

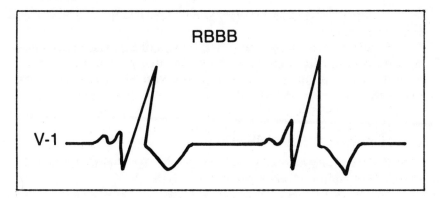

Figure 7.13A. Abbreviation: RBBB = right bundle branch block.

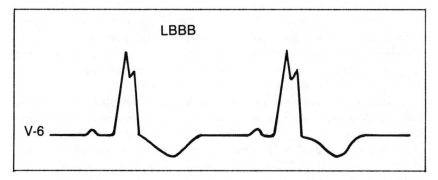

Figure 7.13B. Abbreviation: LBBB = left bundle branch block.

3) LBBB + slowed conduction through the right bundle.

It is difficult to establish the evidence for the slowed conduction through the remaining fascicle. The surface ECG may have a prolonged PR interval or the PR interval may be normal. In order to conclusively establish the diagnosis, one must record the conduction time across the AV node/His–Purkinje system and determine if it is prolonged (His bundle recording). Right atrial pacing or certain drugs (especially procainamide) may uncover a conduction delay where it previously was normal.

Bundle branch blocks and hemiblocks require no specific treatment unless there is evidence suggesting progression to complete heart block.

PREEXCITATION SYNDROMES

Preexcitation is the term used to indicate the ventricle is excited prior to the time it would be excited by normal AV node conduction. This preexcitation is accomplished by bypassing the AV node.

Wolf–Parkinson–White Syndrome

The Wolf-Parkinson-White syndrome (see Figure 7.14) is an electrocardiographic syndrome consisting of:
1) Short PR interval (less than 0.12)
2) Delta wave
3) Wide QRS (more than 0.10 sec)
4) Paroxysmal tachycardias

The anatomical cause of the WPW syndrome is an accessory fibromuscular bundle (Kent bundle) which bridges the gap between the atrium and ventricle thus providing the pathway for the preexcitation of the ventricle. These accessory pathways may be found at virtually any site of the AV border. The *delta wave*, an initial (30 to 50 msec) slow component of the QRS complex, is caused by activation of ventricular myocardium via the accessory connection.

Several other conditions are known to be associated with WPW, including Ebsteins anomaly of the tricuspid valve, mitral valve prolapse and cardiomyopathy.

Tachycardias associated with WPW may be of three types:

1) The incidence of *atrial fibrillation* seems to be increased. When this occurs the atrial impulse may pass down either the normal AV node pathway or down the accessory pathway. If the refractory period of the accessory pathway is very short, it may conduct virtually all of the atrial impulses producing a rapid irregular ventricular rhythm which is unstable and may deteriorate into ventricular fibrillation.

In some patients, *digitalis* may result in shortening of the refractory period of the accessory pathway, consequently the drug is *contraindicated in this condition*. There are also preliminary reports that *verapamil* may do the same and should thus be used with caution (4).

2) *Orthodromic accessory pathway tachycardia* is the most common tachycardia associated with WPW. The tachycardia path-

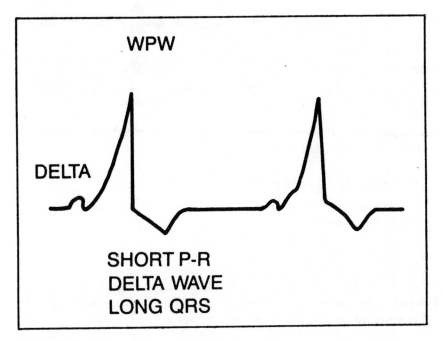

Figure 7.14.

way consists of a reentrant loop with the antegrade pathway comprising the AV node and retrograde loop the accessory pathway. Because the antegrade impulse passes down the normal conduction pathway of the AV node, there is no delta wave on the surface ECG. This type of supraventricular tachycardia is suspected when the ECG reveals an inverted P wave long after the QRS (long R-P/P-R ratio).

3) *Antidromic accessory pathway tachycardia* is less common. The reentrant pathway consists of antegrade conduction down the accessory pathway (resulting in the appearance of a delta wave) and retrograde conduction up the AV node. This tachycardia results in a wide QRS complex and may be mistaken for ventricular tachycardia.

Treatment

Treatment of the tachycardias associated with WPW may be successful with several anti–arrhythmic agents including: procainamide, quinidine, digitalis, propanolol, disopyramide, verapamil and amiodarone. However, the effect of each agent on the refractory period of the accessory pathway is unpredictable.

Digitalis especially (and possibly verapamil [4]) may shorten the refractory period of the accessory pathway resulting in dangerous rapid antegrade conduction. This risk constitutes an important reason for electrophysiologic study in these patients.

In this study, the refractory period of the accessory pathway is determined after the administration of each drug and the best drug for each patient is selected.

Lown–Ganong–Levine Syndrome

Another preexcitation syndrome is Lown–Ganong–Levine syndrome. It consists of:

1) Short PR interval (less than 0.12 sec)
2) Normal QRS duration
3) Frequent paroxysmal arrhythmias

This syndrome is considered to be the result of a James bypass tract which bypasses the AV node and connects to the distal portion of the AV node or His bundle.

The tachycardias associated with LGL are usually reentrant supraventricular tachycardias with antegrade and retrograde pathways being made up of the bypass tract and AV node, respectively.

ANTI-ARRHYTHMIC AGENTS

Quinidine, procainamide, propranolol, and diphenylhydantoin each tend to decrease automaticity of Purkinje fibers. These agents have been divided into two groups on the basis of their different effects on conduction velocity. Quinidine and procainamide decrease membrane conductance and thus conduction velocity in the Purkinje fiber (group I anti-arrhythmic agents); licodaine and diphenylhydantoin either do not change conduction velocity or increase it (group II anti-arrhythmic agents). Quinidine and procainamide then are examples of group I anti-arrhythmic drugs; lidocaine and diphenylhydantoin are examples of group II anti-arrhythmic drugs.

Quinidine

Following a single oral dose of quinidine, gastrointestinal absorption is almost complete. Peak blood levels are reached in

2-3 hours with residual measurable levels for 12-24 hours. The halflife of quinidine sulfate in aterial blood is approximately 6 hours. In persons over 60 years of age, it may exceed 9 hours, thus a corresponding reduction in dosage may be necessary in elderly subjects. At the end of the oral dosage interval of 6-8 hours, the serum level should be 1.5 to 3 mg/liter. Drug levels are usually drawn at the expected peak level (1½ hours after the last dose) and at the lowest level, the trough (just before the next dose). Quinidine sulfate is usually administered orally in doses of 200-600 mg every 6 hours. Initial dose of 600-900 mg daily is suggested. The dosage is then adjusted according to blood levels and anti-arrhythmic efficacy.

The more common toxic effects of quinidine are impaired hearing, tinnitus, diarrhea, and nausea. There is a long list of other reported toxic effects and any significant reaction should warrant discontinuing the drug and substituting another agent in order to determine if quinidine is the culprit.

Procainamide (Pronestyl)

Procainamide is quickly and nearly completely absorbed in the gastrointestinal tract. Peak plasma levels occur within 1 hour after an oral dose and then decline at a rate of 10-20% an hour; 60% of the drug is excreted in the urine. The usual therapeutic range of blood levels is 4-8 mg/liter. The usual oral procainamide dose is 500 mg and is given every 4 hours because of a short half-life. A sustained release form of procainamide has recently become available, and the dosing interval may then be extended, however, this should be guided by blood levels and anti-arrhythmic efficacy.

Procainamide may produce gastrointestinal complications, including anorexia, nausea, vomiting, and diarrhea. Intravenous administration may produce hypotension, myocardial depression, AV block, bundle branch block and ectopic beats. A majority of patients taking the drug for a period of 3 months or longer develop changes in the blood similar to those occurring in patients with lupus erythematosus, including positive LE cell preparations and antinuclear antibodies. A few of the patients develop fever, arthritis, pericarditis, pleurisy, and other features resembling the syndrome of systemic lupus erythematosus. Lupus nephritis does not develop following procainamide therapy but fatal arteritis may. For these reasons, long term treatment with procainamide must be followed closely and the drug discontinued at the first sign of any of the above side effects.

Disopyramide Phosphate (Norpace)

Disopyramide has group I anti-arrhythmic action, similar to procainamide. An oral dose of disopyramide is 80% absorbed from the gastrointestinal tract. Its plasma half-life is approximately 6 hours, with a range of 4-10 hours. The half-life is significantly prolonged when renal function is impaired. A dosage of 150 mg given orally every 6 hours yields a steady-state plasma level in most patients.

Side effects of disopyramide are most commonly related to the anticholinergic activity of the drug. Dry mouth, urinary retention, constipation, dizziness, and blurred vision may occur. In patients with poorly compensated left ventricular dysfunction, hypotension may occur.

Lidocaine

Lidocaine is effective in the management of ventricular premature beats and ventricular tachycardia, especially in the setting of acute myocardial infarction. Given intravenously the maximum electrophysiologic effects occur within 30 sec. Because of rapid redistribution and metabolism, lidocaine must be given frequently or by continuous intravenous infusion following an initial intravenous loading dose of 50-100 mg. If the loading dose is effective, a continuous infusion of 1-4 mg/min in the average 70 kg patient should then be started.

Toxic effects of lidocaine result from its action on the central nervous system. Muscular fasciculations and convulsions, stupor or circulatory collapse may occur. Because the drug is metabolized by liver microsomes, patients with liver disease should be given smaller doses and patients in heart failure should have lower continuous infusion rates because of the decreased liver perfusion.

Diphenylhydantoin

Diphenylhydantoin is both an anti-convulsant and an anti-arrhythmic and is particularly effective in managing arrhythmias associated with digitalis toxicity.

Diphenylhydantoin is absorbed slowly but completely from the gastrointestinal tract. Peak drug levels occur 12 hours after administration of a single oral dose, and steady-state plasma levels occur in 5 to 15 days during chronic oral administration.

The liver is the major route of excretion. The half-life of diphenylhydantoin varies with the plasma level. The half-life is 20 to 25 hours at therapeutic plasma levels and prolonged at higher plasma levels. The half-life is reduced by the concomitant administration of coumadin, butazolidin, isoniazid, phenothiazine and phenobarbital.

The effects of diphenylhydantoin on the action potential duration and effective refractory period (ERP) resemble those of lidocaine. It shortens the duration of the action potential to a greater extent than it shortens the ERP. The net effect is that premature impulses will occur at more negative membrane potentials resulting in a more rapid velocity of conduction (dv/dt) and improved conduction. It also decreases the automaticity of cardiac tissue.

Diphenylhydantoin is the drug of choice for treating supraventricular arrhythmias arising from digitalis toxicity (paroxysmal atrial tachycardia with block). It is also useful in treating ventricular arrhythmias associated with digitalis, cardiac surgery, or general anesthesia. Adverse effects include hypotension and sinus arrest when injected intravenously. The drug's toxic effects on the central nervous system include diplopia, dizziness, vertigo, nystagmus, ataxia, drowsiness, and cerebellar dysfunction. Other toxic effects are skin reactions, Stevens–Johnson syndrome, gingival hyperplasia, pseudolymphoma and megaloblastic anemia.

Beta Blockers

The beta blockers are reversible antagonists of catecholamines at the beta receptors of tissues. Propranolol is the principal beta blocker used clinically in the United States for management of rhythm disorders.

Propranolol's pharmacokinetics are complex and dependent on dose and the duration and route of administration. Propranolol is almost completely absorbed from the gastrointestinal tract, but bioavailability with oral administration is reduced by the first-pass effect in the liver. This is especially true of the initial dose. With chronic oral administration, the hepatic enzyme system becomes saturated and propranolol's bioavailability increases. The drug is matabolized largely by the liver. The initial half-life following an intravenous injection of propranolol is 10 minutes. There is a second half-life of 2-3 hours and anti-arrhythmic effects usually last several hours after intravenous injection.

The electrophysiologic effects caused by propranolol are predominantly the result of blockage of catecholamine effect on cardiac tissue. Consequently the beta blocker inhibits the effects of catecholamines. The results are: decreased automaticity of the SA node (decreased heart rate); decreased conduction velocity and repolarization in the AV node (decreased AV node conduction). At pharmacologic concentrations, propranolol appears to prolong ventricular refractoriness. However, at very high concentrations, propranolol shortens the action potential duration. This effect, which is similar to that of lidocaine, is of questionable importance in the clinical setting.

Propranolol is effective against a broad spectrum of supraventricular and ventricular arrhythmias; it is effective in terminating and preventing atrial premature contractions, paroxysmal atrial fibrillation and flutter, and paroxysmal supraventricular tachycardia. This is especially true if these arrhythmias are related to sympathetic excess during exercise or emotional stress. It also slows the ventricular response rate in chronic nonparoxysmal atrial fibrillation or flutter. Its adverse effects include the production of decompensation in patients with congestive heart failure or chronic obstructive pulmonary disease. It may increase sinus node dysfunction and AV block. It can aggravate peripheral vascular disease and must be used cautiously in insulin-dependent diabetics, because it disguises the sympathetic-mediated warning symptoms of hypoglycemia.

Bretylium

Bretylium is an anti-arrhythmic drug that has been recently released for the parenteral treatment of life-threatening arrhythmias. It is injected intravenously in an initial dose of 5-10 mg/kg. This may be followed by a second dose in 1-2 hours. The maintenance dose is 5-10 mg/kg IV every 6-8 hours.

Bretylium is extremely effective for the treatment of ventricular arrhythmias. It is indicated for ventricular tachycardia refractory to the more commonly used drugs.

Bretylium may initially accelerate the sinus rate, increase the frequency of ventricular premature contractions, and cause hypertension during its initial action, because it causes the transient release of norepinephrine. Later, it can cause hypotension by adrenergic blockade. Nausea and vomiting are also seen.

Verapamil

Verapamil is a papaverine derivative whose major action is as a calcium channel antagonist. It directly affects the SA node and the conduction through the AV node. Its major clinical use is in the termination and treatment of paroxysmal supraventricular tachycardias (including reentrant AV junctional tachycardia, reentry involving an accessory pathway, atrial flutter and fibrillation).

Intravenous doses are 5–10 mg injected slowly. Orally effective doses are 40–80 mg every 8 hours.

Verapamil may cause sinus arrest or bradycardia in patients with sinus node dysfunction, may worsen heart block in patients with underlying AV node disease, and may depress ventricular function in patients with preexisting myocardial disease.

Table 7.3 lists the usual anti-arrhythmic agents and dosages.

Experimental Agents

In addition to the above approved agents, there are several anti-arrhythmic agents which are currently undergoing clinical testing.

Amiodarone is an agent originally developed as an anti-anginal agent, but it has been shown to be an effective anti-arrhythmic agent for the acute and chronic management of supraventricular and ventricular arrhythmias. It has a very long half-life and a low toxic–therapeutic ratio.

Tocainamide is an oral analogue of lidocaine.

Mexilitine is another oral lidocaine-like agent.

REFERENCES

1. Hoffman B, Rosen M, Wit A: Electrophysiology and pharmacology of cardiac arrhythmias. III. The causes and treatment of cardiac arrhythmias. Part A. *Am Heart J, 89:*115-122, 1975.

2. Wit A, Rosen M, Hoffman B: Electrophysiology and pharmacology of cardiac arrhythmias. II. Relationships of normal and abnormal electrical

activity of cardiac fibers to the genesis of arrhythmias. B. Reentry. Section 1. *Am Heart J, 88:*664-670, 1974.

    3. Brugada P, *et al.*: Identical QRS complexes during atrial fibrillation with aberrant conduction and ventricular tachycardia. The value of a His bundle recording. *PACE, 6:*1057-1061, 1983.

    4. Prystowsky E, Prystowsky M: Drug treatment of supraventricular tachycardia in patients with WPS syndrome. *Drug Therapy*, 109-125, December, 1983.

TABLE 7.3
ANTI-ARRHYTHMIC AGENTS

Agent	Indication
Digitalis	SVT (especially atrial fibrillation with rapid ventricular response)
Quinidine	Atrial fibrillation PACs PVCs VT
Procainamide	Atrial flutter PACs PVCs VT
Propranolol	SVT Digitalis-induced tachyarrhythmias
Diphenylhydantoin	Digitalis-induced tachyarrhythmias
Verapamil	SVT Atrial fibrillation
Bretylium	VT V-fib
Tocainide (Lidocaine-like)	PVCs VT
Mexilitine (lidocaine-like)	PVCs VT
Atropine	SB SA block
Isoproterenol	SB AV block
Epinephrine	Asystole

Abbreviations: SVT = supraventricular tachycardia; VT = ventricular tachycardia; PAC = premature atrial contraction; PVC = premature ventricular contraction; V-fib = ventricular fibrillation; SB = sinus bradycardia; AV = atrioventricular; SA = sinoatrial.

Chapter 8

DISEASES OF THE DELIVERY SYSTEM
(Vasculature)

DISEASES OF THE AORTA

Supravalvular Aortic Stenosis

Supravalvular aortic stenosis is stenosis of the aorta just above the valve. Blood pressure is often different in the two arms. There are two varieties of the disease, one is familial, and the other variety is associated with a characteristic facies which consists of widely spaced teeth, dental malocclusion, full cheeks, elfin-like faces, pug nose and a wide mouth with pouting lips. Mental deficiency is usually present, and there is often a history of infantile hypercalcemia.

Coarctation of the Aorta

Coarctation of the Aorta at the Aortic Isthmus. This condition results in hypertension in the upper extremities and low blood pressure and delayed pulse in the femoral arteries. A murmur may be heard over the back of the chest. Approximately 50% will have a bicuspid aortic valve and 10% will have aortic insufficiency. Chest x-ray may show bilateral notching of the inferior margin of the ribs between the 3rd and 10th ribs. This notching is produced by dilation of the enlarged intercostal arteries which carry increased collateral flow.

Marfan's Syndrome

This heredofamilial disorder is associated with cystic medial necrosis of the aorta. There may be associated arachnodactyly (long fingers and toes), increased height, ectopia lentis, hypermobile joints and mitral valve prolapse. The aortic lesion may produce dissection of the aorta, rupture of the aorta and aortic insufficiency.

121

Arteriosclerotic Aortic Aneurysm

These aneurysms are most common in the abdominal aorta, usually originating below the renal arteries and are most frequently in men over the age of 50 years. The aneurysm may be originally found on x-ray of the abdomen showing calcification in the walls of the aneurysm. Radiopaque contrast aortography is necessary to identify the full extent of the aneurysm but CT scan and ultrasound may give valuable clues to its extent. Surgery of the aneurysm is generally recommended when it reaches 6 cm in diameter.

Traumatic Aortic Disease

The sudden deceleration as in a fall or auto accident may result in damage and dissection of the aorta. The portion most vulnerable is that lying just beyond the origin of the left subclavian artery in the thorax.

Syphilitic Aortitis

Syphilis may result in an aortitis of the ascending aorta. It is a late lesion of syphilis occurring 10-30 years after the initial infection. The resulting aneurysm tends to rupture eventually, therefore surgical resection is warranted. Serologic tests for syphilis may be misleading. The Kahn serologic test may be negative in as many as 23% of patients with syphilitic aortitis. The VDRL test is positive in 98-99% of such patients but may be negative in patients over 65 years of age. The Treponema pallidum immobilization test may be positive when the VDRL test is negative and is especially useful when the patient is over 65 years of age or has had antisyphilitic therapy.

Dissecting Aneurysm of the Aorta

This disease is most common in men of middle age with a background of hypertension but is also found in the setting of Marfan's syndrome, cystic medial necrosis, or coarctation of the aorta and is more common in pregnancy. It has also been described in certain heritable disorders of connective tissue, including Ehler-Danlos syndrome and has been observed as a complication of relapsing polychondritis. Approximately 50% of aortic dissections begin in the ascending aorta. A dissecting aneurysm may extend proximally to involve the aortic valve area, thus causing aortic valvular insufficiency; it may extend along the carotid sheath to cause hemiplegia. It may involve the blood supply to the spinal cord, leading to paraplegia and anesthesia below the level of involvement. It may involve the renal artery thus aggravating preexisting arterial hypertension.

Most dissecting aneurysms are associated with chest pain, which may radiate into the abdomen or into the back. Systemic hypertension may be present. Some patients have significant differences of pulse and blood pressure in the arms, legs of carotid arteries. On chest x-ray, a change in the width of the aorta, especially involving the aortic arch, is very suggestive of dissection or of mediastinal bleeding. Aortography is usually required to make the diagnosis.

Treatment of aortic dissection may be either medical or surgical. Surgical resection is recommended when there is continued leakage from a dissection, when the process involves the ascending aorta or arch, when the cerebral circulation is compromised, with severe heart failure caused by aortic regurgitation, when there is evidence of continued dissection, or when pain and blood pressure cannot be controlled.

The medical management of aortic dissection involves control of hypertension and administration of drugs to lessen the systolic ejection force of the heart.

Takayasu's Syndrome

This disease is a form of arteritis which appears, most commonly, in females in Japan. It may affect the aortic arch, the entire arch and its branches or the descending thoracic and abdominal aorta. Symptoms are determined by the area of involvement but may include angina pectoris, dizziness, syncope, headaches and impaired vision with claudication in the upper or lower extremities. Aortography will show extensive stenosis of occlusion and localized aneurysms. Adrenal corticosteroids are the most common form of treatment.

DISEASES OF THE PERIPHERAL VESSELS

Arteriosclerosis Obliterans

This disease is the leading cause of obstructive arterial disease of the extremities after age 30. The lower extremities are involved most commonly. The superficial femoral artery is affected by stenosis or obstruction in approximately 90% of patients. The next common sites are the aortoiliac and popliteal areas.

The most common presenting symptom is intermittant claudication, consisting of cramping pain, tightness, numbness or severe fatigue in the muscles supplied by the affected artery. The amount of exercise producing pain is relatively constant in each patient, and the pain is relieved promptly at rest. If pain begins to occur at rest, this is a grave sign indicating that the blood supply is inadequate even for the small nutritional requirements of the skin.

Diminished or absent pulses will be demonstrated distal to the site of obstruction in the region of claudication. Exercise may be required to bring on the claudication and the decrease in pulse. On auscultation a bruit may be heard over the site of the stenotic lesion. Other signs of ischemia include coldness of the extremity, pallor, cyanosis, rubor and trophic changes. Indolent ulceration and gangrene indicate severe local ischemia.

Lerich's syndrome results from isolated aortoiliac disease, producing intermittant claudication of the low back, buttock, thigh or calves. Impotence may also be present. All pulses are usually absent in the legs, but weak femorals may be felt if the collateral circulation is well developed or if the stenosis is incomplete.

Treatment of intermittant claudication is usually conservative. The patient is advised to exercise frequently to the development of pain but to rest until the pain totally disappears. The aim of this exercise is to open collateral blood vessels. If the claudication is found to be progressively worse or if ischemic symptoms such as numbness or parethesis are present, surgery is considered. Vasodilator drugs, despite wide advertisement, have no significant place in the treatment.

Thromboangiitis Obliterans (Buerger's Disease)

An obliterative vascular disease, inflammatory in type, afflicting chiefly the peripheral arteries and veins. The disease is more common in males, and there is usually a history of cigarette usage.

Young smoking male who presents with evidence of peripheral vascular insufficiency and thromphlebitis. The most frequent presenting complaint is persistent coldness of the limbs. In contraindication to arteriosclerosis obliterans 70% of the patients have involvement of the upper extremities in addition to the lower extremity. Arteriography demonstrates a characteristic lesion.

The treatment is the same as for arteriosclerotic obliterans. Tobacco usage must be stopped. Bilateral preganglionic sympathectomy has been advocated for prominent vasospasm.

Arterial Embolism

Emboli may originate from mural or valvular thrombi in the left side of the heart or from an atheromatous ulcer in the aorta. Paradoxical emboli originate from venous thromboses, travel to the right side of the heart, and pass through a patent foramen ovale. Emboli lodge at bifurcations of arteries and at narrowed arteriosclerotic areas.

Sudden onset of severe pain in the extremity distal to the site of obstruction. Loss of distal pulses, palor, collapsed veins, decreased reflexes and sensation and weakness of the extremity are found. Arteriography is required to confirm the diagnosis.

Embolectomy is the treatment of choice. Awaiting this, treatment should be instituted to improve blood flow including anticoagulation with heparin and possible thrombolytic therapy with streptokinase.

Raynaud's Phenomenon and Disease

A syndrome characterized by paroxysmal, bilateral ischemia of the digits induced by cold or emotional stimuli and relieved by heat.

Demonstration of evidence of ischemia or the fingers on exposure to cold (well demarcated blanching of the fingertips; with recovery, a bright red reactive hyperemia occurs). Trophic changes may occur and the fingers may become thin and tapering with smooth skin, and loss of mobility.

Unsatisfactory but vasodilators are occasionally successful. Sympathectomy may be of benefit in selected cases.

Other Diseases

Acrocyanosis – a vasospastic disturbance of the smaller arterioles.

Ergotism – a vasospastic disturbance due to toxicity of drugs or bread made from rye or wheat infected with ergot fungus.

Erythromelalgia – paroxysmal bilateral vasodilatation of the feet associated with burning pain, increased skin temperature and redness of the skin.

Immersion foot – due to prolonged exposure of the extremity in water.

Frostbite – due to freezing of tissues resulting in damage to skin, muscle, blood vessels and nerves. Treatment should consist of immediate rewarming.

Arteriovenous fistulas – abnormal communications between arteries and veins, resulting in shunting of blood rapidly into the venous circulation. May result in pain, edema, varicosities, hypertrophied extremities or heart failure. A diagnostic sign is Branham's sign (temporary compression of the artery supplying a fistula decreases the heart rate).

PERIPHERAL VENOUS DISEASE

Thrombophlebitis and Phlebothrombosis

The presence of a thrombus in a vein is referred to as phlebothrombosis. An inflammatory reaction may be incited resulting in thrombophlebitis. Predisposing factors include venous stasis associated with constricting garments, severe obesity, postoperative states, congestive heart failure and hemiplegia. Other clinical conditions associated with an increased incidence include ulcerative colitis, malignancies of all types (especially of the pancreas), homocystinuria and prolonged administration of estrogens.

Superficial thrombophlebitis is not difficult to diagnose, because the thrombosed vessel can be felt beneath the skin as a tender cord. Deep vein thrombophlebitis is more difficult to diagnose because there may be no local signs. Helpful diagnostic tests and clues are:

1) Increased circumference of the limb.

2) Homan's sign (pain in the calf and/or popliteal space on dorsiflexion of the foot).

3) Positive cuff test (discomfort in the distribution of the veins on inflating a blood pressure cuff above the site of inflammation).

4) Noninvasive studies of Doppler ultrasonic flow studies and impedance plethysmography are said to be positive in the majority of patients.

5) Ascending radio-contrast venography is the most specific test, but is expensive and carries some risks.

6) Radiolabelled fibrinogen I-125 is another diagnostic test but is not commonly employed because of the risk of hepatitis and the expense.

The treatment of deep vein thrombophlebitis is bed rest, local anti-inflammatory measures and systemic anti-coagulation until the inflammation has subsided.

Varicose Veins

Distended tortuous veins with incompetent valves. These dilated veins may be complicated by thrombophlebitis and afterwards result in chronically swollen extremity due to chronic venous stasis.

Retrograde flow of blood past incompetent valves can be demonstrated by the Trendelenburg test and its variations. The leg of the recumbent patient is elevated to empty the veins, and then a tourniquet is applied to occlude the superficial veins. The patient quickly assumes a standing position, and the tourniquet is released, and the veins will become distended immediately if back flow is present.

Treatment consists of elastic support or bandages. Vein stripping is a last resort.

SYSTEMIC ARTERIAL HYPERTENSION

Prevalence

Approximately 1/8 of the U.S. population (25-30 million individuals) have a diastolic BP of greater than 95. One third of these people have diastolic pressures consistently greater than 105. Another 15 million individuals have "borderline" elevation of blood pressure in the range of 140/90 to 159/94. And it is estimated that only 50% of those with elevated blood pressure that should be under therapy, know they have high blood pressure. Of those with known hypertension, 50% are under treatment, and only 50% of these individuals are being effectively treated.

Symptoms and Complications

Extensive actuarial data supports the concept that life expectancy decreases as blood pressure increases. These are not subtle differences, and they are not dependent only on marked elevation of blood pressure — a 35-year-old male, for instance, with a sustained blood pressure of 150/100 has a life expectancy 17 years less than that of a normotensive cohort.

Symptoms definitely ascribable to hypertension are rare and are generally seen only in malignant hypertension which may present with headache, visual disturbances, seizures, nausea, vomiting, or mental status changes.

We are primarily interested in treating hypertension to prevent the complications of long standing elevated blood pressure, and these are:

1) Congestive heart failure
2) Renal failure
3) Stroke
4) Accelerated atherosclerosis resulting in premature coronary artery disease, peripheral vascular disease and cerebrovascular disease.

When Should Hypertension be Treated?

In general, individuals with a diastolic pressure greater than 90 on three different occasions, taken in the absence of obvious stress are labelled as hypertensive. Marked elevations of the diastolic pressure, in the range of 120-140 should be treated immediately and hospitalization might be recommended if associated symptoms are present or if the diastolic pressure is above 140.

The cutoff for the systolic pressure is 140 to 150 mm Hg, at least in young and middle aged people. Older individuals with isolated systolic hypertension present several problems:

1) Though such hypertension is associated with an increased rate of cardiovascular and renal disease, the elevated blood pressure may be an *effect* rather than a *cause* of arterial pathology,

2) Treatment in this situation is often problematic because of the difficulty in maintaining adequate cerebral perfusion, and

3) These patients may be beyond the point where lowering of the blood pressure positively affects their lifespan.

SECONDARY SYSTEMIC ARTERIAL HYPERTENSION

Over 95% of people with hypertension do not have an identifiable etiology of their elevated blood pressure. Table 8.1 lists treatable causes of secondary hypertension.

An exhaustive search for these causes of hypertension would be too expensive. A standard work-up should include:

1) History and physical examination (will identify such conditions as coarctation of the aorta, Cushings, renovascular hypertension if bruit present)

2) Urinalysis (identify renal disease)

3) Serum electrolytes (identify hypokalemia associated with the mineralocorticoid disorders [Aldosteronism, DOC excess, licorice ingestion])

4) Serum creatinine (evaluates renal function)

5) Electrocardiogram (identifies end-organ damage, i.e., hypertrophy or infarction)

6) Chest radiograph (identify hypertrophy of heart)

7) SMA-12 screening chemistries (will identify hypercalcemia, liver disease, other end-organ damage)

8) CBC (identify polycythemia and other medical illnesses).

The major cause of secondary hypertension which may not be detected by the above tests is renovascular hypertension. This should be suspected in the young (less than 35 years old) hypertensive who is unresponsive to the usual treatment, or with a flank bruit, or absence of a family history of hypertension. This possibility should be evaluated by a rapid sequence intravenous pyelogram (IVP) or renal scan and stimulated plasma renin activity.

A pheochromotoma is a rare cause of hypertension, but it is curable and may not be diagnosed by the above tests. It may produce paroxysmal hypertension, but more commonly, the elevated blood pressure is sustained. It may result in dramatic symptoms of catecholamine excess, or it may be relatively asymptomatic, especially in the familial variety. When it is suspected, it must be investigated with urine and serum tests (catecholamines, metanephrines, VMA).

Treatment of Hypertension

A "Step-Care" approach to the treatment of hypertension is used. This means that initially a drug with a very low probability of side-effects is used. These first-line drugs are either thiazide diuretics or beta-blockers. If the response to this treatment is inadequate, then the thiazide and beta-blocker are combined. If the response is still inadequate then a second-line agent is added. These are: methyldopa, clonidine, prazosin, hydralazine, and reserpine. In the event of still inadequate response, a third line agent is added (minoxidil or captopril).

Figure 8.1 illustrates this simplified approach to treatment.

Hypertensive Emergencies

Hypertensive emergencies include accelerated or malignant hypertension, hypertensive encephalopathy, marked hypertension with acute left ventricular failure or cardiac ischemia, dissecting aortic aneurysm, intracranial hemorrhage, eclamplia and pheochromocytoma crisis.

Drugs used in hypertensive emergencies include: sodium nitroprusside, trimethaphan, diazoxide, hydralazine and reserpine.

TABLE 8.1

- Renal parenchymal disease
- Renovascular disease
- Endocrine diseases
    - Acromegaly
    - Hypothyroidism
    - Cushing's syndrome
    - Aldosteronism (mineralocorticoid excess [licoricel])
    - Hyperparathyroidism (hypercalcemia)
- Coarctation of the aorta
- Increased intracranial pressure
- Polycythemia vera

TREATMENT OF HYPERTENSION

A. CLASSIFICATION OF ANTIHYPERTENSIVE DRUGS
    1. Diuretics
            Thiazides (chlorthiazide, hydrochlorothiazide)
            Loop diuretics (furosemide, ethacrynic acid)
            Potassium sparing (triampterene, spironolactone)
    2. Sympatholytics
            Central action (clonidine)
            Peripheral action (guanethidine)
            Central and peripheral action (reserpine, methyldopa)
            Receptor blockers (phentolamine, phenoxybenzamine,
               propranolol)
    3. Vasodilators
            Atrial action (diazoxide, hydralazine, minoxidil, praxosin)
            Arterial and venous action (nitroprusside, nitroglycerin)

B. EMPIRICAL TREATMENT (STEPPED CARE)
    STEP 1   Thiazides
    STEP 2   add propranolol
               or methyldopa
               or clonidine
               or reserpine
    STEP 3   add hydralazine
               or prazosin
    STEP 4   Loop diuretic + Beta-blocker + minoxidil

Figure 8.1.

Chapter 9

DISEASES PRESENT FROM BIRTH
(Congenital Heart Disease)

The severe and complex anomalies usually are repaired in infancy or result in death. These will not be dealt with here. Only those defects which allow survival to adulthood will be considered. These lesions may be complicated by heart failure, peripheral emboli, and bacterial endocarditis, consequently the general physician and allied health personnel must be familiar with their manifestations.

CAUSES

These include *genetic* (the incidence of congenital heart disease in siblings is extremely high when consanguinity is present), *viruses* (rubella, coxsackie, and mumps), *drugs* (thalidomide, antitumor agents), and *hypoxia.* The risks of a malformed heart resulting from maternal rubella is 40-80% within the first weeks of conception and remains at 25-60% at the tenth week. The most common defects associated with maternal rubella are: Patent Ductus Arteriosus, 58%; Ventricular Septal Defect, 18%; and Atrial Septal Defect, 7%.

COMMON CONGENITAL HEART LESIONS

In the adult the most common congenital heart lesions are:

Atrial Septal Defect. 37%
Coarctation of the Aorta. 16%
Ventricular Septal Defect 12%
Pulmonary Valvular Stenosis. 11%
Patent Ductus Arteriosus. 10%
Tetralogy of Fallot 5%
Valvular Aortic Stenosis 4%

Atrial Septal Defect

This relatively common defect results in shunting of blood from the left atrium to the right atrium resulting in volume overload of the right ventricle. A pulmonary flow murmur is heard at the upper left sternal border and the second heart sound is widely split and "fixed," meaning that the splitting does not change with respiration (Figure 9.1).

Because of the increased shunt flow through the lungs, a chest x-ray shows enlargement of the right ventricle and signs of pulmonary overcirculation.

The EKG characteristically shows a pattern of incomplete right bundle branch block (IRBBB) with rSr' pattern in aVr and V-1 (Figure 9.2).

The M-Mode echocardiogram is helpful in making the diagnosis of an ASD, showing volume overload of the right ventricle (Figure 9.3).

The ASD may be complicated by pulmonary hypertension which causes the shunt to reverse, resulting in cyanosis. Other

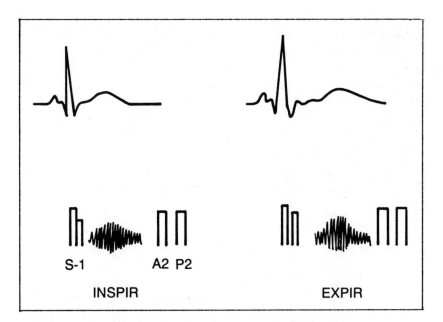

Figure 9.1. Abbreviations: INSPIR = inspiration; EXPIR = expiration.

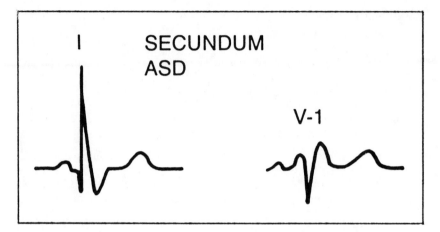

Figure 9.2.

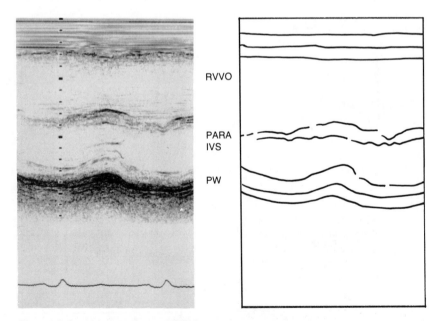

Figure 9.3. Abbreviations: RVVO = right ventricle volume overload; PARA IVS = paradoxic septum motion; PW = posterior wall.

complications include right heart failure, atrial arrhythmias (fibrillation and flutter), and endocarditis.

Surgical closure of the ASD is the treatment of choice and is very effective and of low risk. It results in a lowering of the mortality and risk of complication and should be considered if the volume of left to right shunt is *greater than two to one.*

Coarctation of the Aorta

This condition consists of a congenital narrowing of the aorta, usually just below the left subclavian artery. It will result in hypertension of the upper extremities of 20 mm Hg or greater with its attendant complications.

Reduced or absent femoral pulses point to coarctation. Chest x-ray reveals what is called a "reverse 3 sign" which is a prominent aortic arch, an indentation at the site of coarctation and a bulging of the aorta below the coarctation. Also notching of the inferior portion of the ribs may be present and caused by the dilated collateral intercostal vessels.

Surgical treatment is warranted for significant coarctation.

Ventricular Septal Defect

VSD is the most common congenital cardiac anomaly in infants. It is seen only occasionally in adults, because if not corrected in infancy, it carries a high mortality. In addition, many of the small defects close spontaneously in childhood.

In infancy the VSD may result in pulmonary hypertension and congestive heart failure, but in adults, because the defect is usually very small, these complications rarely result.

On examination one hears a harsh systolic murmur along the left sternal border. The pulmonic second heart sound may be prominent if the shunt flow is large. Gallop sounds may be present if congestive failure supervenes.

Chest x-ray may reveal signs of pulmonary over-flow and ECG may indicate ventricular hypertrophy, right or left, depending on the direction of the shunt. Surgical closure is usually undertaken to prevent infective endocarditis.

Pulmonary Valvular Stenosis

See chapter five.

Patent Ductus Arteriosus

This condition is rarely seen in adults, since it is usually corrected in childhood. The characteristic physical finding is a continuous machinery-like murmur heard at the first and second left intercostal space and radiating to the back. The murmur envelopes the second sound with late systolic accentuation and terminates in late or middiastole (Figure 9.4).

The chest x-ray shows left ventricular and left atrial enlargement, and the pulmonary artery may be dilated and the lung fields may show increased flow. The ECG is normal in a small ductus but will show left ventricular hypertrophy with a large shunt. In a large defect with a large shunt, the left atrium will be dilated and the degree of this dilatation correlates with the degree of shunt.

Surgical correction of the PDA is warranted for prevention of bacterial endocarditis.

Tetralogy of Fallot

This is the only common cyanotic heart disease in the adult. The entity was described by Etinne-Louis Arther Fallot in 1888 and consists of a ventricular septal defect, pulmonary stenosis

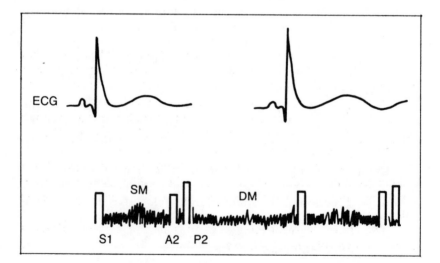

Figure 9.4. Abbreviations: SM = systolic murmur; DM = diastolic murmur.

(valva or infundibular), overriding of the aorta and right ventricular hypertrophy. The essential anatomic components producing the pathophysiology of right-to-left shunting with cyanosis are the ventricular septal defect and pulmonary stenosis.

Squatting is a frequent activity of the child with "Tet," because this increases systemic resistance and decreases right-to-left shunting thereby improving oxygenation.

On auscultation an aortic ejection click, ejection systolic murmur and single second sound (A-2) are present. Occasionally aortic regurgitation is present and an immediate diastolic murmur is noted. The ECG characteristically shows right axis deviation and right ventricular hypertrophy. On the chest x-ray, the heart has a characteristic "boot shape" with reduced pulmonary blood flow and diminished lung vasculature. There is a concavity in the region of the pulmonary trunk and a prominent aortic arch, which is frequently right-sided. Collateral pulmonary blood flow may come from bronchial vessels.

Previously, shunt operations (Blalock-Taussig, Potts-Smith-Gibson, Waterson, and Brock operations) were usually performed to improve pulmonary blood flow. However, the technique of total correction has become well established. Successful surgery decreases the risks of the complications of infective endocarditis, cerebral thromboembolism, and brain absess.

Valvular Aortic Stenosis

Aortic valvular stenosis that occurs as an isolated lesion is a nonrheumatic disorder resulting from either of two disease processes. One process is progressive calcification and stenosis of a congenitally abnormal valve — usually a bicuspic aortic valve or sometimes an unicommissural or mildly stenotic tricuspid aortic valve. Calcification and stenosis of a congenitally abnormal valve is the most frequent cause of calcific aortic stenosis in patients less than 60 years of age. The other process involves degenerative thickening and calcification of leaflets in originally normal valves, which is the most frequent cause of calcific aortic stenosis in elderly patients.

The clinical and diagnostic features are those discussed in the chapter on valvular heart disease.

Chapter 10

MISCELLANEOUS CONDITIONS (Endocarditis, Pericarditis, Pulmonary Heart Disease)

INFECTIVE ENDOCARDITIS

Infective endocarditis is a microbial infection implanted on a heart valve or on the wall of the endocardium. Four mechanisms are responsible for the initiation and localization of the infection:

1) A previously damaged cardiac valve or a hemodynamic situation in which a so-called jet effect is produced by blood flowing from a zone of high pressure to one of relatively low pressure, as in mitral insufficiency or ventricular septal defect;

2) a sterile platelet-fibrin thrombus;

3) bacteremia, often transient; and

4) a high titer of agglutinating antibody for the infecting organism.

Normal hearts are only rarely the seat of subacute endocarditis. The commonest situations for its development are chronic rheumatic heart disease and congenital heart disease. Acute endocarditis is commonly seen in previously normal hearts.

Table 10.1 shows the usual sites of the endocarditis lesions in the various cardiac conditions.

A Venturi effect is produced when blood is driven from a high pressure source through an orifice into a low pressure sink, explaining the distribution of lesions complicating various cardiac valvular and septal defects. Turbulence and the jet effect traumatize the endothelial surface and initiate a plate-fibrin thrombus which may lead to the establishment of an infected focus. Transient bacteremia occurs frequently in normal persons and these bacteria adhere to the sterile platelet-fibrin thrombus. This adherence is aided by circulating antibody to the organism, especially agglutinins. By clumping the organisms, the antibody

TABLE 10.1
SITES OF ENDOCARDITIS

Condition	Sites of Endocarditis
Coarctation of Aorta	Downstream aorta
Patent ductus arteriosus (PDA)	Pulmonary artery
A-V fistula	Communicating veins
Ventricular septal defect (VSD)	Right ventricle surface of defect
Aortic insufficiency (AI)	Ventricular surface of aortic valve
Mitral regurgitation (MR)	Atrial surface of mitral valve
Pulmonic insufficiency (PI)	Ventricular surface of pulmonary valve
Tricuspid insufficiency	Atrial surface of tricuspid valve

produces an inoculum large enough to induce multiplication and infection.

Pathoanatomic, Pathophysiologic and Clinical Correlations

Four mechanisms are involved in the development of the clinical features of infective endocarditis.

The Infectious Process of the Involved Valve

This is responsible for:
1) Constitutional reactions (fever, malaise, weight loss, anemia)
2) Changing heart murmur
3) Leukocytosis
4) Destruction of cardiac structures (tears, aneurysms, congestive heart failure)

Embolization

Except for congestive heart failure, arterial emboli are the most frequent complications of infective endocarditis. The most common sites are the coronary vessels, spleen, kidneys, and brain.

Metastatic Infections and Mycotic Aneurysms

In the acute type of infectious endocarditis, especially that caused by Staphylococcus aureus, infection is frequent at sites of embolic deposition. These metastatic infections are rare when Streptococcus viridans and other relatively noninvasive organisms may result in myocardial abscesses, cerebral abscesses as well as infection of other organs.

Mycotic aneurysms are a major complication of infective endocarditis but are frequently undetected before autopsy. These lesions are most frequent when relatively noninvasive organisms such as Streptococcus viridans are involved and less common when the causative agent is Staphylococcus aureus.

Immunologic Aspects and Hypersensitivity Phenomena

Agglutinating, complement-fixing and opsonizing antibodies that are specific for the infecting organism are regularly present in patients with infective endocarditis, especially the subacute form.

These Result In: Rheumatoid factor, increased IgG and IgM levels, high concentrations of cryoglobulins and macroglobulins, immune-complex glomerulnephritis, and vasculitis (resulting in Osler's nodes, Janeway lesions, Roth spots, subungual hemorrhages and petechiae).

Organisms Involved: A recent study reported the following organisms as most commonly involved:

Viridans streptococci.	34%
Staphylococcus aureus	25%
Enterococci.	6%
Other streptococci.	14%
Diptheroids	4%
Staphylococcus epidermis	3%
Other bacteria	7%
Candida albicans	2%
Culture negative	5%

Endocarditis following cardiac surgery is usually caused by a Staphylococcus, often coagulase negative. (Therefore, growth of Staphylococcus epidermis from a blood culture must be considered important and not written off as a contaminant.)

Blood Cultures: Bacteria are discharged from valvular vegetations at a relatively constant rate independent of the patient's temperature. In subacute endocarditis, when immediate empiric therapy is not necessary, two cultures a day for 3 days ordinarily suffice. In acute endocarditis, when the patient is so ill that empiric therapy cannot be delayed, three cultures at half-hour intervals should be made and therapy then instituted.

Endocarditis Involving the Right Heart: Currently, adult drug addicts with right-sided vegetations on the tricuspid valve are seen with great frequency. These infections are characterized by: 1) a high frequency of pulmonary infarct or abscess, 2) a lower incidence of positive blood cultures, and 3) a higher incidence of cases in which murmurs are not heard.

Treatment

In the choice of antibiotics for the treatment of endocarditis, one should refer to the current literature on the specific organisms. Some guidelines are:

Viridans streptococci: Two treatment regimens are generally used for subacute bacterial endocarditis due to penicillin-susceptable strep of the viridans group. The first employs aqueous penicillin alone in doses of 2-12 million units per day for 4-6 weeks. Equally good results (95% cure) are achieved when penicillin is combined with streptomycin and administered for 4 weeks.

Enterococcus: The recommended therapy for enterococcal endocarditis is the combination of penicillin or ampicillin in large daily intravenous doses (10-30 million units per day) plus intramuscular streptomycin (500 mg every 12 hours). Treatment should be continued for 6 weeks.

Staphylococcus aureus: The duration of antimicrobial therapy of Staphylococcus aureus endocarditis should be 6 weeks. Intravenous penicillin (10-20 million units per day) is the drug of choice if the organism is a nonpenicillinase-producing Staphylococcus. With Staphylococcus resistant to penicillin, a penicillinase-resistant penicillin should be used.

Prophylaxis against endocarditis: Transitory bacteremia may be caused by a variety of manipulations or surgical procedures, and in the individual with structural heart disease, such bacteremia may initiate endocarditis. Certain procedures are associated with a high risk of bacteremia such as: dental extraction (60-90%) and transurethral prostatic resection (10-60%). Antibiotic prophylaxis is recommended in the following procedures: dental procedures, surgery of the respiratory tract (e.g., tonsillectomy), procedures of upper respiratory tract (e.g., bronchoscopy), surgery or instrumentation of the genitourinary tract (including urethral catheterization), surgery and instrumentation of the lower gastrointestinal tract and gallbladder, obstetric infections (e.g., septic abortion or peripartum infection), cardiac surgical procedures requiring extracorporeal circulation, and surgical procedures on infected or contaminated tissues.

Specific treatment regimens are recommended by the American Heart Association, and these should be consulted for each specific circumstance.

PERICARDIAL DISEASES

There are three major pericardial diseases: acute pericarditis, pericardial effusion and constrictive pericarditis.

Acute Pericarditis

This condition is an acute inflammation of the pericardium. It is usually idiopathic, although it is assumed to be of viral origin. There are several other conditions which may cause pericarditis. Some of these are:

1) Connective tissue disorders (rheumatic fever, scleroderma, rheumatoid arthritis, lupus erythematosis, Takayasu's arteritis, polyarteritis nodosa, Wegener's granulomitosis)

2) Uremia

3) Acute bacterial infection

4) Trauma

5) Tuberculosis

6) Fungus infections (Histoplasmosis, Blastomycosis)

7) Radiation

8) Neoplasm

9) Drugs (hydralazine, procainamide, INH, penicillin, phenylbutazone)

10) Protozoal infections (amebiasis, Toxoplasmosis)

11) Miscellaneous infections (actinomycosis, Reiter's syndrome, echinococcal disease, psittacosis–lymphopathia venereum group, mycoplasm)

12) Miscellaneous (sarcoidosis, myxedema, amyloid, myeloma, acute pancreatitis)

13) Delayed post–myocardial infarction (Dressler's syndrome), post-pericardial injury syndrome

The clinical features of acute pericarditis consist of chest pain, a characteristic friction rub and an abnormal ECG.

The precordial pain of acute pericarditis is usually of a sharp nature and tends to be accentuated by deep breathing, lying down and rotating the trunk. Often it is relieved to some extent by sitting up and leaning forward.

The pericardial friction rub is found in only 70% of patients with acute pericarditis. Most typically it has three phases: one associated with atrial systole, one with ventricular systole, and one with ventricular diastole. Often, however, there are only two phases: one associated with ventricular systole and one with diastole. If a pericardial friction rub cannot be readily heard, the patient should be examined in several different positions, including recumbency, sitting upright and even in the knee–chest position.

The ECG of pericarditis is related to inflammation or injury of the myocardium which lies just beneath the epicardium. The characteristic feature of early acute pericarditis is elevation of the S-T segments, which is greatest in the leads where the QRS complex is upright, so that the elevation is usually present in II and occasionally in III of the standard leads and in most of the precordial leads. It is often absent in lead V1 and usually absent in lead aVr. As the pattern of pericarditis evolves, the S-T segments tend to return to the baseline. This may occur within a few hours or a few days. The T waves in acute pericarditis may become negative after the S-T segments return to the baseline. Figure 10.1 shows a lead from a characteristic ECT of acute pericarditis.

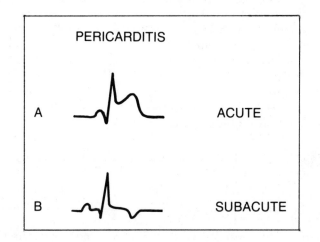

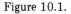
Figure 10.1.

The ECG of acute pericarditis must be differentiated from that in *acute myocardial infarction* and the normal variant pattern of *early repolarization.* The ECG of acute MI usually shows reciprocal depression of S–T segments and has pathologic Q waves. The early repolarization pattern usually occurs in young males, most frequently blacks. As a rule, the ST segment changes in early repolarization are not as widespread as in acute pericarditis, and the T wave is more likely to be normal. The best way to distinguish the two is by serial ECGs. In acute pericarditis, a change in ST–T contour may be expected within a few days.

The treatment of acute paricarditis consists of relief of symptoms and the treatment of the underlying systemic illness. In idiopathic nonspecific pericarditis, reassurance, bed rest as long as fever and pain persist and asprin for relief of pain are usually all that are required. When the disease is clearly unrelated to a specific viral, fungus, bacterial or protozoal disease and pain is unrelieved by salicylates, the administration of cortocosteroids may produce dramatic results. After initial high dose steroid therapy, the drug is tapered over the following 6-9 weeks. When steroid therapy cannot be withdrawn without recurrence of symptoms, pericardial resection or azathioprine therapy may be indicated.

Pericardial Effusion with Tamponade

Acute pericardial tamponade occurs when fluid accumulates rapidly in the pericardial cavity, compressing the ventricle and restricting ventricular filling. This may be caused by:
1) Idiopathic pericarditis
2) Neoplastic disease
3) Uremia
4) Rupture of the ventricle after myocardial infarction
5) Dissecting aortic aneurysm
6) Collagen vascular disease
7) Trauma

Clinically, cardiac tamponade is characterized by elevated venous pressure (in severe cases there may be an actual increase in venous pressure during inspiration = Kussmaul's sign), narrow arterial pulse pressure, abnormal fall of blood pressure on inspiration (greater than 10 mm Hg), known as paradoxic pulse, and tachycardia. On chest x-ray one sees a rapidly enlarging cardiac silhouette with clear lungs. In patients with pericardial effusion, there is often decreased voltage of QRS and T complexes on the ECG. Electrical alternans may be present.

The echocardiogram is clearly the superior diagnostic instrument for pericardial effusion, as echo-free spaces being demonstrated around the heart. Figure 10.2 demonstrates an M-mode echo showing a pericardial effusion.

Pericardiocentesis is usually reserved for therapy of severe tamponade and not for diagnostic purposes because of the inherent risk involved.

Constrictive Pericarditis

Constrictive pericarditis occurs when visceral and parietal pericardial layers become fused, thickened, densely fibrotic and

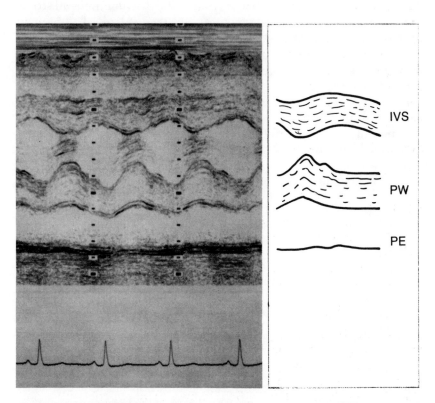

Figure 10.2. Abbreviations: IVS = interventricular septum; PW = posterior wall; PE = pericardial effusion.

inelastic and form a rigid case around the heart. The pericardial space is obliterated and calcification may occur. In a particular patient, the cause may be unknown (idiopathic) but often the cause is among the following:

1) Infection (viral, bacterial, tuberculous, fungal)
2) Collagen vascular disease
3) Neoplasm
4) Trauma
5) Radiation

The clinical features of this condition develop gradually and include:

1) Failure to transmit changes in intrathoracic pressure to the intrapericardial spaces; and

2) Limitation of ventricular filling by fibrous encasement. Because of limited ventricular filling, ventricular end-diastolic, atrial, and jugular venous pressure rise, while stroke volume and cardiac output are reduced.

Gradual compensatory changes in the peripheral circulation may help to maintain blood pressure despite diminished cardiac output.

As in the normal ventricle, ventricular pressure decreases rapidly during early diastole. However, rapid ventricular filling occurs only during a brief interval in early diastole before the limit of ventricular distensibility is reached. As rapid filling occurs, the pressure tracing displays an abnormally abrupt rise and a high late diastolic plateau, commonly referred to clinically as the "square root sign." End-diastolic pressure may exceed 1/3 of systolic pressure. An audible "pericardial knock" often accompanies early diastolic filling and is attributed to vibrations produced by the sudden deceleration of blood as it strikes the encased ventricular wall. Figure 10.3 illustrates the "square root sign" with equalization of end-diastolic pressures of the right and left ventricles.

In the patient with constrictive pericarditis, the pulmonary wedge pressure (reflecting mean left atrial and left ventricular end-diastolic pressures), pulmonary arterial diastolic pressure all tend to be equal, since the heart is encased in a common rigid chamber. The decrease in vena caval pressure associated with inspiration is absent. Occasionally, in severe cases there may be an actual increase in venous pressure during inspiration (Kussmaul's sign). This sign probably reflects increased intra-atrial pressure occurring when the adherent pericardium is pulled taut as the diaphragm descends.

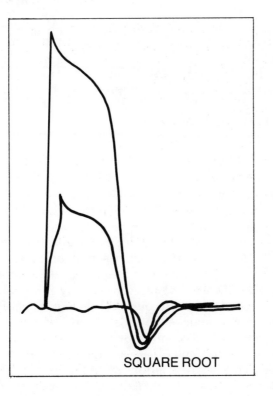

SQUARE ROOT

Figure 10.3.

Symptoms in constrictive pericarditis may include effort dyspnea, chest pain, right upper quadrant or epigastric pain, effort syncope, orthopnea and paroxysmal nocturnal dyspnea.

There is an intermediate form of constrictive pericarditis that runs a more rapid course and is often associated with pericardial effusion, as well as with pericardial fibrosis and myocardial constriction. This disorder has been called *effusive-constrictive pericarditis.* Patients with this disorder may develop cardiac constriction within a matter of several months. There is considerable pericardial effusion as well as pericardial thickening.

The treatment of constrictive pericarditis is influenced by its severity and its known or suspected causes, as well as its duration. When constrictive pericarditis is mild, not disabling, and slowly progressive, surgical resection of the pericardium may be postponed for years, or indefinitely. When the process has progressed rapidly in a matter of months, effusive–constrictive pericarditis may be present and respond to corticosteroid therapy. Surgical pericardial resection should be considered in patients with severe disease and limiting symptoms. Relative contraindications to surgical resection include: old age or presence of other major illness; heavy calcification of the pericardium, the presence of evidence of significant myocardial involvement.

PULMONARY HEART DISEASE

The normal mean pulmonary arterial pressure in man, dogs and other mammals averages 15 mm Hg, with a range of 12-17 mm Hg. As the blood passes through the lungs, the pressure falls so that by the time the blood reaches the left atrium, the mean pressure is 2-12 mm Hg. If the average pulmonary arterial pressure is assumed to be 15 mm Hg and the average left atrial pressure is 9 mm Hg, the difference of pressure in only 6 mm Hg across the pulmonary vascular bed. Because of the low pulmonary arterial pressure in normal man, elevations of left atrial pressure such as may occur with mitral stenosis or left ventricular failure cause a significant increase on pulmonary arterial pressure.

A physiologic classification of pulmonary hypertension is:
1) Passive (elevation of pulmonary venous pressure)
2) Hyperkinetic (increased pulmonary blood flow)
3) Obstructive (pulmonary embolism or thrombosis)
4) Obliterative (reduction of pulmonary vascular capacity)
5) Vasoconstrictive (functional vasoconstrictive reaction)
6) Polygenic (arising in one or more of the above ways)

Often more than one mechanism is involved in human pulmonary hypertension. For example, in chronic obstructive airway disease, hypoxia and respiratory acidosis may cause vasospastic pulmonary hypertension, pulmonary fibrosis and vascular intimal proliferation may cause obliterative pulmonary hypertension.

Cor Pulmonale

Cor pulmonale is defined as hypertrophy of the right ventricle resulting from disease affecting the function and/or the structure of the lung except when these pulmonary alterations are the result of diseases that primarily affect the left side of the heart or of congenital heart disease.

The most common background for cor pulmonale is that of chronic obstructive airway disease, causing more than 50% of the cases of cor pulmonale in the U.S. Other conditions known to cause cor pulmonale are:

1) Pulmonary vascular obstructive disease
   a. Pulmonary thromboembolism
   b. Idiopathic pulmonary hypertension
   c. Sickle cell anemia, especially hemoglobin SC disease
   d. Bilharziasis
   e. Pulmonary hypertension of high altitude
2) Pulmonary granulomatous disease
   a. Berylliosis
   b. Sarcoidosis
3) Pulmonary fibrosis
   a. Bronchiectasis
   b. Pneumoconiosis
   c. Radiation
   d. Scleroderma and other collagen vascular disorders
   e. Idiopathic pulmonary fibrosis, including Hamm–Rich syndrome.
4) Miscellaneous pulmonary disease
   a. Alveolar proteinosis
   b. Idiopathic pulmonary hemosiderosis
   c. Congenital cystic disease of the lung
   d. Bronchopulmonary dysplasia related to respirator therapy and oxygen intoxication.
   e. Gaucher's disease
5) Chest wall disease
   a. Kyphoscoliosis
   b. Rheumatoid spondylitis
   c. Thoracoplasty
6) Neuromuscular disease
   a. Muscular dystrophy
   b. Poliomyelitis
   c. Amyotropic lateral sclerosis
7) Hypoventilation states
   a. Primary respiratory center hyposensitivity to carbon dioxide.
   b. Obesity hypoventilation (Pickwickian)
   c. Hypoventilation associated with enlargement of tonsils and adenoids

8) Mucoviscidosis
9) Chronic mountain sickness
10) Pulmonary dysmaturity (Wilson–Mikity syndrome)

Heart Failure

Patients with long standing respiratory insufficiency often develop heart failure manifest as elevated venous pressure and peripheral edema. Right ventricular failure is well established as a complication of chronic pulmonary disease, while left ventricular failure is controversial, it may also occur in the later stages of chronic respiratory insufficiency.

If cor pulmonale occurs in a patient with chronic obstructive airway disease, it usually appears after some 5–10 years or more of symptomatic chronic obstructive airway disease. In the stage before heart failure, cor pulmonale is seldom recognized clinically. Its appearance is suggested by ECG or x-ray evidence of right ventricular enlargement. However, the ECG changes may be difficult to distinguish from those of chronic obstructive airway disease alone, and the roentgen evidences of right heart enlargement in COPD are seldom striking. Heart failure in cor pulmonale with COPD is usually evidenced by the onset of dependent edema.

ECG

The ECG in cor pulmonale of COPD may show right axis deviation of P and QRS with predominantly S waves across the precordium. There may be P pulmonale and "lead I" sign (P and QRS are almost invisible in I). Atrial arrhythmias, including atrial fibrillation, atrial flutter or chaotic atrial rhythm are common.

Heart Catheterization

In severe lung disease and cor pulmonale, arterial pressure is increased above the normal of 12–17 mm Hg. The pulmonary wedge pressure, reflecting pulmonary venous pressure, is usually in the normal range of 6–12 mm Hg. The right ventricular systolic pressure is increased and equals pulmonary artery systolic pressure, but the diastolic pressure is usually normal unless the right ventricle fails. Then the right ventricular diastolic pressure and right atrial pressure rise above the normal range of 0–5 mm Hg to as high as 20–25 mm Hg.

Treatment

In treating patients with cor pulmonale, primary attention should be directed towards improving the pulmonary function; treatment of congestive heart failure is a secondary target. Thus, one first treats pulmonary infection, bronchospasm, hypoxia and respiratory acidosis and then congestive heart failure when it is present.

When there is congestive heart failure, this may be treated as in other varieties of heart disease. Sodium intake should be restricted and diuretics instituted. Digitalis preparations may be employed in cor pulmonale with heart failure because it increases cardiac output, but must be used cautiously, especially when patients are undergoing correction of respiratory acidosis where potassium may shift intracellularly, increasing the danger of digitalis–related arrhythmias. Digitalis is also useful in patients with atrial flutter, atrial fibrillation or paroxysmal atrial tachycardia and multifocal atrial tachycardia.

Chapter 11

AGING AND THE
CARDIOVASCULAR SYSTEM

It is projected that by the year 2000, there may be 50 million people in the U.S. over the age of 65. This expanding part of the population has unique health care problems which must be addressed and solved. The majority of diagnosed and treated heart disease will be in this elderly population, and the majority of the population which survives to this age will have some degree of heart disease. Additionally, because of sensitivity to medication, complications of treatment are more likely in the elderly than in the young.

The commonest cause of death and disability in the elderly population is heart disease. There are various common manifestatins of heart disease seen in this age group, and the medical student, nurse, and physician should be familiar with them and their complications.

CONGESTIVE HEART FAILURE

Congestive heart failure (CHF) is an extremely common disorder in the elderly and is most commonly due to hypertension or coronary artery disease and, according to some studies, perhaps due somewhat to the aging process itself. The manifestations are those discussed in the chapter on congestive heart failure: shortness of breath and swelling of the feet and ankles. The elderly may not be aware of shortness of breath but notice that they have difficulty lying flat, and the observation by others that respiration is rapid (greater than 20 per minute) may be the only clue. The usual treatment consists of digitalis preparations (digoxin, digitoxin, etc.) diuretic agents (which promote salt and water excretion), and a salt-restricted diet.

Complications of the Disease in the Elderly

Because of accumulation of fluid in the lungs, these patients are vulnerable to the development of pneumonia. Influenza is particularly dangerous and life-threatening; they should receive the appropriate vaccine against influenza, and, in treatment, should receive amantadine (an antiviral agent). Because of the immobility associated with CHF, venous stasis and deep vein phlebitis often develop in the veins of the lower limbs, bringing the risk of pulmonary embolism (clots to the lungs). This is a life-threatening complication and may be subtle with only an acute shortness of breath, chest pain and coughing up of blood.

Complications of Treatment

Complications of treatment of CHF in the elderly include digitalis toxicity and fluid and electrolyte depletion. The elderly are particularly prone to digitalis toxicity because of decreased lean body mass, the storage depot of digitalis, and decreased renal function, leading to accumulation of the drug in the body. This must be suspected when there is a loss of appetite, yellow vision or other visual disturbances, irregularities of heart beat and ultimately disorientation and delirium. Diuretics will cause depletion of the body potassium leading to muscle weakness and fasciculations and heart rhythm irregularities. Seriously low blood potassium may be a life-threatening situation and should be aggressively searched for with blood samples and should be treated promptly. Use of diuretics along with severe fluid restriction may result in serious fluid depletion and dehydration, consequently the patient should be weighed daily so as not to have to precipitate a loss of fluid.

CORONARY ARTERY DISEASE

The chapter on coronary artery disease deals with this condition more fully. The manifestations may consist of angina pectoris (chest pain — classically, a squeezing sub-sternal sensation which may be brought on or worsened by exertion), myocardial infarction (heart attack), and cardiac rhythm irregularities. Unfortunately, the elderly may not complain of chest pain either because of lack of perception due to drugs or decreased mental acuity or damage to pain-transmitting nerve fibers from other diseases (e.g., diabetes mellitus). A sudden deterioration in well-being may be the only clue to the development of one of these conditions. Symptoms may include those of congestive heart failure, palpitations and syncope.

Complications of the Disease

Complications of the disease include congestive heart failure, cardiogenic shock and life-threatening cardiac irregularities including ventricular tachycardia and ventricular fibrillation. If these are suspected, arrangements must be promptly made for heart rhythm monitoring and appropriate pharmacologic treatment.

Complications of Treatment

Complications of treatment for coronary artery disease may also occur. Nitrates and beta blocking agents are commonly given for the management of angina pectoris. Nitrates are frequently prescribed in long-acting forms and may cause hypotension. Beta blocking agents may mask the signs of hypoglycemia in the insulin dependent diabetic, and may produce congestive heart failure in the patient with significant pre-existing heart damage. Because none of these agents are without potentially serious side-effects, patients taking them must be closely followed in order to detect significant changes in the effects of the drugs.

HEART BLOCK

Heart block is considered in more detail in the chapter on cardiac rhythm disturbances, but it occurs of sufficient frequency in the elderly to require special consideration. There are several varieties of heart block with different degrees of seriousness and significance. Milder forms include First degree block, and Second degree of Mobitz I. These usually do not produce syncope and are not life-threatening. Mobitz II Second degree heart block and Third degree heart block (complete heart block) are life-threatening, produce syncope and must be promptly recognized and treated. Temporary hemodynamic support may be possible with drugs such as atropine and isoproteronol, however, the definitive treatment is a demand intra-cardiac pacemaker. A temporary pacemaker may be inserted via a peripheral vein pending arrangement for a permanent implant.

Complications of the Treatment

Complications of the treatment are unusual but may occur. These include rupture of the ventricle in which the pacing electrode is placed, run-away pacemaker in which the generator suddenly begins to drive the heart very rapidly, battery failure in which the generator fails, and failure to sense in which the pacemaker fails to sense the patient's intrinsic heart beat and discharges inappropriately, producing additional arrhythmias.

ANEURYSM

This is a balloon-like dilatation of an artery. An aneurysm may occur almost anywhere, but the major problems are with aneurysms of the aorta, either in the chest or the abdomen. In the chest the aneurysm usually shows up as an enlargement of the ascending aorta shadow on the chest x-ray. In the abdomen an aneurysm may be a pulsating mass that is perceived by the patient but is usually first noted by the physician on examination. There may be no symptoms associated with an aneurysm unless the bulge is involving other body organs. If the aneurysm is expanding, there is usually pain and this may be severe, consisting of a ripping, tearing variety. Complete diagnosis of an aneurysm requires CT scanning and/or arteriography. Treatment of this life-threatening condition requires surgery, and this must be considered urgently if the aneurysm is enlarging.

Complications of the Treatment

Complications of the treatment include occlusion of other arteries being supplied by the aorta, or embolism of clot from the repaired site. The patient should be observed for serious cold feet, sudden pain in one or both legs, discoloration of the legs or paresthesias (numbness) of distal extremities.

PERIPHERAL VASCULAR DISEASE

This disorder is a particular problem in elderly patients. Gradual narrowing of the arteries occurs to a point where the blood supply becomes inadequate. At first the symptoms may be mild, consisting of pain in the calves on walking and relieved by rest. Later, pain becomes more severe and occurs during rest, particularly at night. A feeling of numbness (paresthesias) and coldness in one or both feet is noted. It may involve only a toe or may include the entire leg. Ultimately, there is death of tissue due to inadequate blood supply, leading to gangrene that results in loss of part of all of the extremity. Complaints of pain or numbness in the feet or legs should arouse suspicion and lead to further investigation. Careful palpation for the distal pedal pulses of the dorsalis pedis and posterior tibial arteries. The patient may have no complaints, yet one observes that a toe or foot is blue and cool to the touch. The problem is extremely common in diabetics so these people require extremely careful foot care with particularly close observation and treatment of minor cuts, abrasions, or infections. Applying heat may be dangerous, since the blood supply cannot be increased to meet the augmented demands because of narrowing of the arteries.

SYSTEMIC HYPERTENSION

Blood pressure tends to rise normally with advancing age, because the peripheral vasculature becomes less compliant so degrees of elevated systolic pressure which would be treated in the younger population is best not treated in the elderly population. Also, if elevated systolic blood pressure is lowered too rapidly in the elderly population, this may decrease brain perfusion and result in somnolence, irritability and confusion. On the other hand, sustained increased blood pressure may produce damage to target organs producing heart failure, coronary artery disease and strokes. Successful treatment definitely lowers the risks of such complications. It appears that appropriate treatment would be lowering of blood pressure gradually so as not to produce serious side effects to the treatment.

Complications of the Treatment

Complications of the treatment of hypertension are those associated with too rapid reduction of blood pressure resulting in decreased cerebral perfusion and stroke, and side effects from the drugs used. Most commonly these are fluid and electrolyted depletion secondary to diuretic treatment. In particular, loss of serum potassium will result in fatigue, weakness, and muscle fasciculations. This must be monitored closely and potassium replacement undertaken as necessary.

STROKES

A stroke is also known as a cerebrovascular accident (CVA). There are several types and several causes, but the net effect is destruction of some part of the brain. These cells lack the capacity to regenerate themselves so the loss is irreversible. One type, the cerebral hemorrhage, is almost always seen in severe hypertensive people and is a dramatic, often lethal event. A cerebral thrombosis, the most common type in elderly people, occurs when a clot forms in one of the arteries to a portion of the brain. The commonest location is an artery that affects pathways to an entire side of the body and face, resulting in partial or complete paralysis of half the entire body. Speech may be completely and irrevocably lost if the dominant side is affected. The stroke may be preceded by transient episodes from which there is complete recovery (called a "transient ischemia attack" = TIA); it is important that these incidents be brought to the attention of a physician since specific measures might be instituted to prevent a final paralyzing event.

The complications of a stroke are those associated with the forced dependence on others and invalidism. These include bed sores, fluid and electrolyte depletion aspiration pneumonia, and malnutrition.

ON DEATH AND DYING

Because one of the major first manifestations of cardiovascular disease in the elderly is death, the health profession must be prepared to deal with the subject, both with the patient and the family. Many who die of cardiovascular disease die suddenly, within an hour of the first symptoms, and this makes for a particularly traumatic experience for the family, especially if the event was unexpected. On the other hand, if the person has a long history of cardiovascular illness, the sudden event may not be unexpected. But the terminal event may still result in serious trauma and anger in the family, therefore the doctor, nurse, and therapist must be prepared to recognize when and where help is needed to cope with the situation.

In interviews with patients with a terminal illness, Kubler-Ross identified five stages through which the patient passed after becoming aware of the prognosis. These stages are:

> First stage: Denial and isolation
> Second stage: Anger
> Third stage: Bargaining
> Fourth stage: Depression
> Fifth stage: Acceptance

The family of a dying person also seems to go through similar stages. Especially in the event of a sudden death, the progress through the stages may be rapid. Denial is the first logical reaction but after being faced with evidence of ambulance, paramedics, emergency room personnel, and our physicians bringing the grim news, the reaction soon progresses to anger. This anger may be largely unfocused at first, then it may become directed towards the patient (e.g., for not heeding prior warnings), the ambulance or emergency room personnel (for not doing all that they could to save the patient), and then to the reporting physician or nurse. The last is one reason that the task of telling the family is frequently given to the lowest doctor on the totem pole. The demeanor of a well-meaning but relatively inexperienced young physician (who is probably bewildered himself over the meaning of the experience) may encourage the anger and resentment as well as the conviction that everything possible was not done. It is imperative here for the professional reporting the terminal event to give the family time to digest the meaning of his words. A blundering, "Well, he bought the farm," is unbelievably crude and unfeeling and can be expected to result in a hostile reaction. It is best to attempt to prepare the family for the eventual announcement by having them notified as early as possible of the seriousness of the sudden illness and to give them some hope yet of recovery. Hope, for even a few minutes, is something that must not be denied to shocked and unprepared spouse and family. Finally, when it is evident to the physician that there is no hope for the patient, the family must be told in a manner which gives them some understanding of the sudden event. It is helpful to briefly go over events and circumstances which led up to the sudden attack, because this approach will often help explain to them the sudden demise. There will be time later for detailed reflection, but the family has some immediate need to put the occurrence into some sort of perspective. The physician must take time to answer questions and try to give some explanation for the suddenness of the event. The door should be left open for future explanations and clarification after the shock of the initial trauma has passed.

In the case of the expected death, the recognition of the stages through which the patient must work, after understanding the prognosis, will help both patient and family to cope with them. In particular, the depression must be recognized and discussed openly. Usually this does not require pharmacologic treatment, but open discussion will frequently help the individual to work through this period.

The health care professional can accomplish much more for the patient if he or she accepts death and dying as a natural consequence of living and can face and guide the adjustment which must be made by the family and patient in preparing for the event and coping afterward.

REFERENCES

1. Kubler-Ross E: *On Death and Dying.* New York: Macmillan Co., 1969.

Chapter 12

WARNING SIGNS OF AN IMPENDING CARDIAC EVENT AND EMERGENCY PROCEDURES

SYMPTOMS AND SIGNS

The major cardiovascular events which the health care professional must be prepared to recognize and manage are:
1) Acute myocardial infarction
2) Acute tachy-or brady-arrhythmia, and
3) Cerebrovascular accident (CVA = Stroke)

There are certain symptoms and signs which should warn one of an impending event, and these should be heeded so that possible preventative action can be taken.

Chest Pain

Many patients with myocardial infarction will have premonitory chest pain similar to angina pectoris although more severe and more prolonged. As described in the chapter on coronary artery disease, the pain may be described as a "tightness," "squeezing," or "pressure" sensation. Most will state that the pain is severe and is frequently associated with sweating (diaphoresis). The sudden onset of severe chest pain in a patient known to have coronary artery disease or at a high risk of coronary artery disease must be viewed with alarm by the health care professional and appropriate action undertaken. Arrangements should be made for electrocardiography and cardiac exam. If these can be performed during the chest pain, one may find evidence of ongoing myocardial ischemia. On the exam this might consist of an S4 gallop or a new heart murmur of mitral regurgitation caused by ischemia of one of the papillary muscles. On the electrocardiogram, this might consist of new ST-T wave changes.

Severe Shortness of Breath

The sudden onset of severe shortness of breath might herald the beginning of a myocardial infarction presenting as acute heart failure with pooling of blood in the pulmonary vasculature. In an acute myocardial infarction, this may occur without associated chest pain. Other causes of acute shortness of breath include pulmonary embolus, respiratory failure of bronchospastic lung disease (asthma), spontaneous pneumothorax, and acute pneumonia. (Although in this condition, the dyspnea usually develops over several hours.)

Palpitations

Palpitations are a common symptom and do not, in and of themselves, indicate probable cardiac emergency. However, if the palpitations are occurring frequently and especially if associated with runs of rapid palpitations ("flutters") with dizziness or a feeling of faintness, they should be investigated. These symptoms may indicate that a significant tachy- or brady-arrhythmia is imminent.

Dizziness, Syncope

Episodes of dizziness and frank syncope may be premonitory signs of more serious impending cardiovascular collapse. Tachy-arrhythmias and brady-arrhythmias, including heart block may result in dizziness and brief spells of loss of consciousness before complete cardiovascular collapse (Stokes–Adams attacks). Certain valvular heart diseases, including aortic stenosis and IHHS, may produce syncope and in these conditions is a particularly ominous prognostic sign.

Transient Ischemia Attack (TIA)

The sudden and temporary onset of a neurologic symptom such as transient facial or limb paresis, slurred speech, blackness appearing in a visual field, may be a premonitory sign of an impending stroke. Suspicion of a TIA should prompt attention and further neurologic evaluation.

Significant Rise or Fall in Blood Pressure

Labile blood pressure should prompt further investigation. A rise in blood pressure may precipitate angina pectoris or may be a result of anxiety from the chest pain. An endless circle may result where anxiety results in higher blood pressure which results in more angina leading to greater anxiety. A significant fall in blood pressure may also be the cause or result of a cardiovascular event. If ischemia of the myocardium is severe then pumping ability may be impaired and blood pressure drop. If the drop in blood pressure is severe enough then coronary perfusion pressure may be significantly decreased resulting in greater ischemia. The cause of the rise or fall in blood pressure must be identified and appropriately managed, otherwise more significant damage may result.

Significant Rise or Fall in Pulse Rate

A sudden drop in pulse rate may indicate a serious brady-arrhythmia or be a premonitory sign of a Stokes–Adams attack, indicating the probability of the development of complete heart block and subsequent syncope. The demonstration of this sign should be followed by an electrocardiogram or cardiac rhythm monitoring in order to more clearly define what the actual problem is.

The finding of a sudden rise in heart rate might indicate that the patient is having serious tachy-arrhythmias, such as paroxysmal supraventricular tachycardia or ventricular tachycardia. If the latter arrhythmia is found on cardiac rhythm monitoring, it should be treated as an acute emergency because ventricular tachycardia is highly predictive of subsequent sudden death. The demonstration of ventricular tachycardia would generally warrant immediate intravenous anti-arrhythmic therapy, continuous cardiac monitoring and transport immediately to an intensive care unit.

MANAGEMENT OF EMERGENCY CARDIAC PROCEDURES

Patients with Acute Myocardial Infarction

Among patients dying suddenly, about 20% have a myocardial infarction. In some, the signs and symptoms develop over several days prior to the terminal event, and a major problem is delay in seeking medical attention because of denial and misinter-pretation of the gravity of the symptoms. This delay in hospitalization and seeking of medical care is a major cause for death following an infarction. About 60% of the sudden cardiac deaths occur within the first hour of onset of symptoms. It will require a superhuman effort at patient education to overcome entrenched fears and habits and educate the public to seek medical aid early after the onset of symptoms.

The physician or other health professional can shorten the delay by advising the patient to proceed immediately to an appropriate health care facility if there is an abrupt onset of chest pain or if preexistent angina pectoris changes in quality or duration. The patient should be instructed to contact an emergency ambulance service directly if symptoms are severe or disabling.

When the health professional is called upon to see a patient having an acute coronary event, the first objective is to allay anxiety and the second is to ease pain. The first requires a reassuring demeanor and encouragement; the second requires parenteral morphine or other major analgesic. The next objective is to protect against fatal arrhythmia-ventricular tachycardia and fibrillation. Monitoring is not required for the initiation of prophylactic anti-arrhythmic treatment with lidocaine. Even in the absence of premonitory ventricular extrasystoles, prophylactic lidocaine may prevent malignant ventricular arrhythmias. The administration of 75 mg. intravenously followed by 300 mg intramuscularly will often prevent these arrhythmias. If symptomatic bradycardia is present and heart rates are less than 50 per minute, the judicious use of small doses of atropine may prove useful, but care must be taken not to produce dangerous over-acceleration of the heart rate. (Doses of 0.5 to a total of 2.5 mg over 2 hours is usually safe and efficacious).

Patients with Primary Electrical Failure

This syndrome usually occurs suddenly without warning and death is frequently nearly instantaneous. The terminal rhythms are:
1) Ventricular tachycardia
2) Ventricular fibrillation, or
3) Bradycardia-asystole

There are two levels of response to this terminal event. The first involves the lay public and all medical personnel and consists of training for cardiopulmonary resuscitation (CPR). The second level involves emergency medical services, emergency physicians and paramedical personnel in training and providing ADVANCED CARDIAC LIFE SUPPORT. This consists of intravenous fluid and drug administration, cardiac defibrillation, stabilization of blood pressure, rhythm monitoring, control of arrhythmias, and post-resuscitation care.

Emergency first aid procedures, consisting of the recognition of airway obstruction and of respiratory and cardiac arrest and the proper application of cardiopulmonary resuscitation (CPR), constitute the elements of BASIC LIFE SUPPORT. CPR involves opening and maintaining a patent airway, providing artificial ventilation by means of rescue breathing, and maintaining artificial circulation by means of external cardiac compression. Paramount among the goals of CPR is to restore a cardiac mechanism as rapidly as possible. The objectives in cardiac resuscitation are the prompt delivery of oxygenated blood to vital organs by means of cardiac massage and the reestablishment of a heart beat by means of defibrillation. If a defibrillator is not at hand then cardiopulmonary efforts are undertaken until the patient can be transported to an appropriate facility.

CARDIOPULMONARY RESUSCITATION

Thump Version

At the very beginning of cardiac arrest, the first arrhythmia may be ventricular tachycardia resulting from a self-sustained reentrant wavefront of depolarization circling around the perimeter of an infarct or an ischemic area. A very low level shock may break the wavefront and terminate the tachycardia. Such low energies can be delivered by a chest thump. Effectiveness of the chest thump is due to transduction of the mechanical input to an electrical pulse, i.e., an abnormal reentrant excitation. One should deliver a sharp, quick blow to the midportion of the sternum, hitting with the lower, fleshy portion of the fist from a distance of 8-12 inches above the chest. It must be administered during the first minute after onset of the cardiac arrest. If there is no cardiac response on repeating the chest thump, cardiopulmonary resuscitation must be instituted.

Artificial Ventilation

The first important feature of successful resuscitation is establishment of a patent airway. This requires examination of the mouth to assure that no obstruction is present such as loosely fitting dentures, vomitus, or any other foreign body. The victim's head should be tilted backwards as far as possible, and this simple maneuver may suffice for the resumption of spontaneous respiration, because the base of the tongue may obstruct the upper airway when the victim lies flat on his back. The head tilt maneuver is accomplished by placing one hand beneath the victim's neck and the other hand on the forehead and then lifting the neck while pressing the head backward. The head must be maintained in this position throughout resuscitation, then mouth-to-mouth or mouth-to-nose breathing is initiated. With one hand behind the victim's neck holding the head in a position of maximum backward tilt, the nostrils are pinched together with the thumb and index finger of the other hand. Next one opens the victim's mouth widely, takes a deep breath, places his mouth over the victim's mouth to create a tight seal, and exhales completely. This cycle must be repeated every 5 seconds for as long as respiratory failure exists. By observing the rise and fall of the chest and by noting the escape of air during exhalation as well as the resistance encountered during inspiration as the victim's lungs expand, the rescuer can determine whether ventilation is adequate.

Artificial Circulation

Cardiac arrest is recognized by the absence of a pulse in the large arteries of an unconscious victim who is not breathing. After rapidly ventilating the victim four times, one next checks for a carotid pulse. If none is felt then external cardiac compression is instituted. The patient should be placed on a hard surface, preferably the floor. Elevation of the lower extremities while the rest of the body remains horizontal may promote venous return and augment artificial circulation during external cardiac compression. The procedure of artificial circulation involves compression of the heart between sternum and spine (Figure 12.1). The pressure required must be of a magnitude to depress the lower sternum by a minimum of 3-5 cm. The long axis of the heel of one's hand is placed parallel to and over the long axis of the lower half of the sternum, while the heel of the other hand is placed on top of the

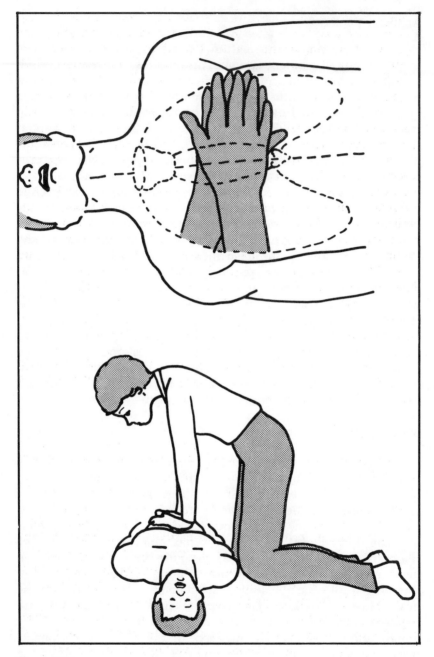

Figure 12.1

other. If applied too high, the massage will prove ineffective and may cause multiple rib fractures. The arms are kept straight at the elbows to allow pressure to be applied almost vertically. The shoulders of the resuscitator should be directly above the victim's sternum so that compression can be carried out by forceful movements of the back and shoulders with elbows fully extended rather than by flexion and extension of the arm at the elbow. Compressions must be regular, uninterrupted, and carried out at a frequency of 60 per minute; relaxation should be abrupt and equal to compression duration. A ratio of 5:1 is maintained between ventilation and cardiac compression.

CPR is best accomplished by two rescuers, one on either side of the victim, who can then switch positions when necessary without any significant interruption of the 5:1 rhythm. If the rescuer is alone, 18 compressions should be applied, and the lungs should be ventilated two times, and this cycle should be continued until help arrives. These points are illustrated in Figure 12.1.

ADVANCED CARDIAC LIFE SUPPORT

Advanced life support refers to the methods and techniques used to supplant basic life support as additional resources and personnel reach the scene.

Supplemental Oxygen

Supplemental oxygen is used to increase the oxygen saturation of the blood being pumped by CPR.

Defibrillation.

Arrhythmia monitoring is preferable during defibrillation, however, if ventricular fibrillation is suspected, blind defibrillation is preferred rather than waste time before gaining an adequate ECG. The electrode paddles to be used must be adequately covered with electrode paste in order to lower electrical impedance. One electrode is placed in the right 2nd intercostal space rather than over the sternum. The other electrode is either placed in the midaxillary line in the 5th intercostal space or, preferably, if a flat paddle is available, positioned posteriorly at the angle of the left scapula. This anteroposterior paddle placement reduces energy requirement by about 50%. When a single discharge fails to convert the arrhythmia, a second discharge at the same energy level will frequently prove successful because of lowering of the skin impedance from the first discharge, thereby delivering more energy.

Intravenous Medications

Once ventilation and cardiac massage have been adequately established several intravenous drugs may be helpful in the resuscitation attempts. If circulation is not restored, sodium bicarbonate (1 mEq/kg) should be injected to reverse metabolic acidosis and is repeated after 10 minutes. Once an effective rhythm is restored, further drug administration is governed by arterial blood gas and pH measurements. Other drugs which may prove useful are:

Epinephrine (0.5 ml of a 1/1000 solution diluted to 10 ml) — used to improve myocardial contractility if there is ineffective myocardial contraction.

Atropine (0.5 to 2.0 mg) — used if there is profound bradycardia.

Lidocaine (75 mg followed by a continuous infusion of 2–3 mg/min) — used to combat premature ventricular contractions and to raise the ventricular fibrillation threshold.

Morphine sulfate (5–8 mg) — used to allay pain and anxiety, especially if pulmonary edema is present because the drug decreases ventricular filling and relieves the edema.

Calcium chloride (2.5–5 ml of a 10% solution) — used to increase myocardial contractility. When calcium gluconate is used, the dose is 10 ml of a 10% solution providing 4.8 mEq of calcium.

Chapter 13

CARDIAC REHABILITATION: A MULTIDISCIPLINARY APPROACH

Following a myocardial infarction or heart surgery, there is frequently a need for physical and psychological rehabilitation. Physical rehabilitation for two reasons: The bed confinement of the illness results in serious deconditioning of the body, and reconditioning prompts faster recovery and decreases the probability of complications from the trauma of the heart attack or surgery. Studies have shown that those patients who are well conditioned suffer fewer complications from hospitalization and surgery than those patients who are in poor condition.

Psychological rehabilitation is warranted because of the emotional trauma of the serious life-threatening illness. Frequently the event of the heart attack or heart surgery is the first time the individual has faced the fact of his or her own mortality and the contemplatation of this with the objective evidence supplied by the hospitalization in an intensive care unit results in serious adverse psychological reactions. Many of these individuals have a personality type (in some studies, designated as a "Type A personality") which is hard-driven and demanding. They are accustomed to being in control of and on top of circumstances around them. They are oriented to "getting things done," of seeing projects to a rapid and successful conclusion. Frequently, however, after a myocardial infarction or heart surgery, they find themselves at the mercy of others — being told by their cardiologist, their husband/wife or their colleagues to "take things easy," to do this or not do that — in essence to relinquish some of the jealously guarded control over his or her own life. One finds himself no longer in control of daily circumstances. Compelled to be waited on by nurses, spouse and family, instructed by doctors and nurses to leave decision-making to others, these patients frequently suffer serious depression and withdraw with bitterness within themselves. Psychological counseling, in concert with the physical and medical conditioning directed by the patient's doctor can greatly help in re-orienting the patient's mental outlook to a more healthy viewpoint. The individual can learn to adjust to the new set of surrounding circumstances and control the self-destructive impulses of temper flares of impatience. A sympathetic counselor can guide the patient through the rehabilitation process and the individual will emerge with a more positive self-awareness and ability to cope with stress and frustration. Evidence would suggest that a psychological adjustment to a more relaxed lifestyle and a less contentious response to frustration may also decrease the individual's risks for subsequent cardiac events.

An example from the author's experience of a patient with a self-destructive reaction to stress was a 27-year-old man who had a heart attack and was hospitalized several weeks for recovery. Prior to the hospitalization he had attempted to keep two jobs and was driving himself relentlessly. The heart attack was complicated by temporary heart block, requiring a temporary pacemaker, congestive heart failure requiring other catheters and complicated procedures. Despite considerable damage to his heart muscle, he survived and was eventually transferred out of the coronary care unit and to his room for recovery. After several days of recovery, I told him one day on rounds that he had recovered sufficiently to allow him to go home the next day. He asked what time he would be able to go, and I casually answered, "About 10 o'clock." The next day I was delayed (as is often the case) and didn't reach his room until 10:15. I found him livid, pacing up and down the floor beating his fist in his hand. When he saw me he exploded, "You said 10 o'clock and you're late! Now I want you to discharge me now and get me out of here!" His blood pressure and pulse must have been tremendously elevated producing a serious stress on his already compromised cardiovascular system. I managed to soothe him and reason with him about the self-defeating nature of his temper. He did leave the hospital but he never returned to me in follow up, seeking, I suppose, a more punctual cardiologist, one who would fit into his schedule.

It was obvious that this young man had learned nothing about his own self-destructive behavior despite the vivid and near-fatal experience of his heart attack.

CORONARY PRONE BEHAVIOR

A behavior pattern which has been shown by Friedman and Rosenman to be related to coronary heart disease is that called

"Type A behavior pattern." This has also been referred to as "coronary prone behavior pattern." It was conceptualized as consisting of six components:

1) an intense, sustained desire to achieve;

2) a profound eagerness to compete;

3) a persistent drive for recognition;

4) seemingly continuous involvement in many activities that were subject to mental and physical functions; and

5) an extraordinary mental and physical alertness.

The 8-year follow up from their study revealed that subjects assessed as possessing the Type A behavior pattern had more than twice the risk of developing clinical coronary heart disease as the subjects originally assessed as non-Type A.

Price has proposed a set of beliefs and fears related to the Type A behavior pattern consisting of certain proposed social and cultural fears, personal beliefs, and personal anxieties:

Social and Cultural Fears: Since upward mobility in an open economy is theoretically unlimited, one will be successful if one tries hard enough. The criteria for success are material accomplishments and related status.

Personal Beliefs: I must constantly prove by my accomplishments that I am successful (worthy of esteem, love and approval). There is no universal moral principle, no orderly (predictable) relationship between the intention of my actions and their consequences. All resources are scarce; therefore, your win is my loss, and I must strive against everyone to get what I need.

Personal Anxieties: Fear of insufficient worth, of being considered unsuccessful. Fear that right actions may produce negative consequences and that wrong actions can produce good consequences (i.e., nice guys finish last).

The essence of the behavior pattern, according to Price, centers around the belief that one needs to prove himself. She discusses how trying to prove oneself can lead to the traditionally accepted characteristics of the Type A behavior pattern and how these characteristics might relate to one another. The belief in the need to prove oneself (often manifested as "unbridled ambition") leads to setting high performance standards. In competition with other hard driving people these antecedents lead to: a chronic sense of time urgency, easily aroused impatience, longer working hours, accelerating pace of ordinary activities, and easily aroused irritability ("free floating anxiety") (1).

Treatment Intervention

Various treatment studies seeking to modify Type A behavior have been reported. Most treatment programs have focused almost exclusively on managing stress and tension without adequate attention to other components of the Type A pattern. It has also proven difficult to measure post-treatment Type A behavior because of the intimate relationship that exists between treatment protocol and assessment measures. Consequently no study to date has proven that the behavior pattern can be modified and that this modification results in a decrease in the coronary risk. Various physiological variables (e.g., cholesterol, triglycerides, heart rate, and blood pressure) thought to be associated with chronic stress have been assessed with differing results. Some studies have reported significant decreases in both serum cholesterol and systolic blood pressure after treatment of the Type A behavior pattern.

At present, a project is underway, "The Recurrent Coronary Prevention Project," to determine to what degree Type A behavior can be modified in patients after they have had a heart attack.

MYOCARDIAL INFARCTION

Early Ambulation

Following myocardial infarction in the early 1900s, it was common practice for physicians to completely immobilize patients for weeks afterwards. It was believed that physical activity would markedly increase the occurrence of ventricular aneurysm and ventricular rupture and, because of the increase in myocardial consumption associated with exercise, increase the risk of arrhythmia, recurrent myocardial infarction and sudden death. This assumption was based on morphologic studies which had showed that it takes 6 weeks for the scar of a myocardial infarction to heal. Also, studies revealed a higher incidence of myocardial rupture among postinfarction patients in mental hospitals than among patients in private hospitals, and it was postulated that this was attributable to the increased activity of mentally deranged patients as compared to the enforced bed rest of the private hospitalized patients.

Levine, in the 1940s, popularized the "chair treatment of acute coronary thrombosis" consisting of allowing the patient to sit in a chair two to three hours a day. This was thought to be beneficial, because it increased peripheral venous pooling, decreasing venous return, and reduced cardiac work. No complications occurred in the first patients reported and an enhanced sense of well-being and easier resumption of activity were also described. Over the 1950s, 1960s, and 1970s the pattern of shortening the period of hospital stay emerged. Studies confirmed that most serious complications of myocardial infarction occur during the first days of hospitalization and that the overwhelming majority of patients with an uncomplicated completed myocardial infarction have little or no in-hospital mortality and very few significant late hospital complications. It has been shown that most patients without continued or recurrent cardiac pain, serious rhythm disorders, cardiac decompensation, or other major complications can safely leave the hospital after the first week or 10 days, consequently this is a common current practice.

Potential for Prevention

The potential for prevention of myocardial infarction and sudden death has been extensively studied for the past several years (see Table 4.3). The probability of death following recovery from myocardial infarction is formidably high as demonstrated by the Framingham study. In this study a cohort of patients from Framingham, Massachusetts were followed over several years. It was found that, following a first myocardial infarction, 20% of men and 45% of women will die within the first and most dangerous year (2). This high post-MI mortality has led to an aggressive approach to the further diagnosis and mangement of these patients. Coronary arteriograms performed early in the posthospital convalescent period may identify the high-risk patient eligible for surgical therapy. The chief determinants of subsequent mortality are:

1) myocardial function (degree of damage from the MI), and

2) coronary anatomy (degree of compromise of the coronary circulation).

Therefore, it is common practice today, even if the patient is asymptomatic, to perform cardiac catheterization and coronary arteriography following MI.

Risk Factors for Early Mortality

Exercise Stress Test

Current practice of management of patients after a myocardial infarction usually includes a low-level stress test. A "positive" or abnormal test, consisting of an ischemic response, significant arrhythmias, or hypotension, usually indicates multivessel disease involving more arteries than those directly producing the infarction.

Persistence of ECG Abnormalities

If the ECG reverts to normal in the following year, the subsequent prognosis is lower than if there are residual ECG abnormalities.

Ventricular Premature Complexes

Ventricular ectopic activity in the recovery stage of a myocardial infarction, particularly if frequent, may indicate extensive ventricular dysfunction and are significant predictors of subsequent sudden death. In patients recovered from a myocardial infarction, ventricular premature complex frequencies of 30 or more per hour are widely considered as definitely dangerous and advanced-grade, multi-form and runs are considered to be even more significant.

Risk of Late Mortality

Traditional coronary risk factors which are correlated with late mortality after an MI are:
1) Systemic Hypertension
2) Hypercholesterolemia
3) Smoking
4) Obesity
5) Diabetes Mellitus

Beta Adrenergic Blockers

Beta adrenergic blocking agents offer promise of reducing postinfarction sudden death. Clinical trials of practolol, alprenolol, propranolol, and timolol suggested that cardiac death following myocardial infarction may be reduced by long-term beta blockade. Benefits may come from reduction in oxygen demand or suppression of ventricular premature beats.

Antiplatelet Drugs

Recently completed trials suggest that administration of antiplatelet drugs (aspirin and dipyridamole) may improve chances of survival after myocardial infarction; however, the results of these trials are inconclusive.

Education and Instruction

Following myocardial infarction, each patient should receive an educational and instructional plan specific for his or her needs. Most patients know that they need to alter their lives after leaving the hospital and are usually awaiting guidelines and instructions. The emphasis in teaching should be *pre*scription and not *pro*scription, i.e., emphasis on "do" rather than overbearing on the "don't." Most patients will react negatively to unmitigated admonitions to change long practiced habits, but will more likely make positive changes if a genuine interest is shown in their welfare and guidelines and encouragement are offered in a nonjudgmental atmosphere.

The Teaching Plan

The following topics should be in the teaching plan.

Coronary Heart Disease: The patient should be informed about his or her disease with specific detail of coronary anatomy and ventricular function and its significance. Coronary risk factors should be discussed with plans laid out to evaluate for and correct those manageable risk factors (serum cholesterol, triglyceride, HDL).

Activity, Exercise, Rest, Work: Specific instructions should be given concerning progressive levels of activity expected, specific types of exercise allowed or prohibited, the amount and time of rest and potential types of work which may be allowed. Education about avoidance of extremes of temperature and humidity should be undertaken. Avoidance of highly competitive leisure activities should be practiced.

Sexual Intercourse: Most patients can resume sexual activity with a familiar partner within four to eight weeks after myocardial infarction. The cardiac work of sexual activity is comparable to that of ascending and descending two flights of stairs or walking briskly. Stress on the cardiovascular system during orgasm, when maximal elevation of heart rate and blood pressure occur, averages 15–20 seconds in duration. If the patient experiences chest pain or discomfort, he can be instructed to take nitroglycerin before intercourse.

Travel: For many patients travel is a way of life and does not necessarily have to be stopped after an MI. Some time must be spent in adjusting to the demanding features of travel and special care and precaution should be undertaken to ensure safety. Prolonged hurried walking with heavy suitcaees must be specifically avoided; the myocardial oxygen cost may be too great resulting in myocardial ischemia. Plan and preparations for adjustments to jet lag and changing time zones must be undertaken, allowing ample time for biologic rhythms to catch up. Jet travel means that a patient will be exposed to oxygen pressure equivalent to that at 4000–5000 elevation and, if there is preexisting hypoxemia, then oxygen supplementation must be undertaken.

Nutrition: Diets should be suggested based on information about fasting serum cholesterol, triglyceride and blood pressure. If the patient is a diabetic, this may also determine certain aspects of the diet. Conceivably, a patient may receive different instructions on restriction of carbohydrate, fats, alcohol, and sodium. Too rigid an approach to nutrition may result in malnutrition and uncooperativeness of the patient. Imagination and individualization must be practiced by the dietician in order to achieve the desired goals. Patients from different ethnic backgrounds should also receive instructions and advice concerning the fat and salt contents of their native foods and the prescribed diets should include foods which are familiar.

Medications: Patients should receive instruction concerning when and how to take their medications. They and a family member should be familiar with the expected effects and potential side-effects of each medication.

Cigarette Smoking: Every reasonable educational effort should be undertaken to encourage the patient to discontinue smoking. The patient needs non-judgmental support from the spouse, family, and health care personnel. Like with alcoholics and weight watchers, the non-smoker role model is most effective in changing addictive behavior habits.

EXERCISE AND THE HEART

Exercise Physiology

Maximal oxygen uptake is an important parameter which is frequently referred to in exercise physiology. It is a stable and highly reproducible characteristic of the individual and serves as a measure of the functional capacity of the cardiovascular system. It is determined by: body size, sex, age, level of regular physical activity, and by a genetic factor. Figure 13.1 illustrates maximal oxygen uptake by age and sex.

In cardiovascular disease, impaired cardiac output may decrease maximal oxygen uptake limiting exercise capacity. Comparison between expected and observed maximal or symptom-

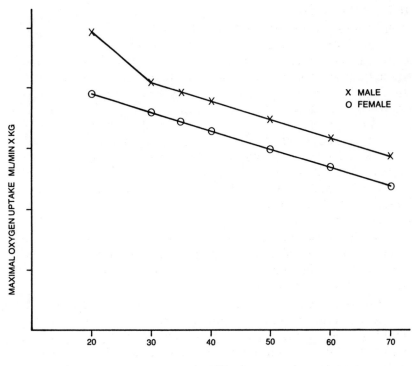

Figure 13.1

limited maximal levels of oxygen uptake may be used to quanti-
tate the functional impact of cardiovascular disease. That is, the
functional significance of heart disease can be quantitated and
followed serially by measuring maximal oxygen uptake. The maximal oxygen uptake does not correlate well with the extent of
coronary artery disease but does reflect the degree of myocardial
damage from the disease.

Exercise Prescription

Frequently, following myocardial infarction or coronary
bypass surgery, a patient wishes to go on an exercise program. This
can be encouraged if the patient's functional limitation from the
disease is not too great. This should be first assessed by a diagnostic exercise stress test, determining what work load the patient can
go to without significant adverse effects (decrease in blood pressure; cardiac arrhythmias; ischemic ST-T changes). After the diagnostic stress test, the physician then knows at what heart rate and
work load a patient develops these significant adverse effects. The
exercise prescription should then incorporate this information,
generally, recommending that the patient exercise to a heart rate
which is 85% of that required to produce these adverse effects.
Time must be taken to teach the patient how to take his or her
pulse properly. If the patient appears to be at significant risk from
arrhythmias, then the initial phase of exercise should be under a
properly medically supervised program.

There are warning signs of excessive effort during or following exercise. These are:

1) Angina discomfort above level 2 on a scale of 1-4.
2) Increased palpitations
3) Inappropriate bradycardia
4) Inappropriate tachycardia during exercise and persistent
tachycardia beyond 6 minutes after exercise
5) Ataxia, light-headedness, confusion
6) Nausea, vomiting
7) Pallor, cyanosis
8) Dyspnea persisting for more than 10 minutes
9) Prolonged fatigue
10) Unusual insomnia afterwards

The target heart rate used in the exercise prescription is a
useful and simple method of following the exercising patient, but

it must not be abused. Recent changes in clinical status, i.e., inter-current illness, anemia, orthopedic injury, etc., should warrant a change in the prescription.

The Role of Health Care Professionals

Physical Therapists make a major contribution to a cardiac rehabilitation program. The in-hospital phase consists of progressively increasing physical activity under the supervision of a physical therapist trained in identifying adverse cardiovascular effects of activity and exercise.

An *Occupational Therapist* also make a major contribution to the cardiac rehab program by providing leisure time activities for the recovering patient and teaching skills and techniques to rechannel energies and frustrations into more constructive channels.

A *Cardiac Nurse* is frequently employed to supervise the in-hospital phase of the program. The nurse should be trained in basic life support procedures, arrhythmia monitoring and recognition techniques, the concepts of myocardial oxygen supply and demand, and in patient education. The nurse is normally responsible for educating the patient about his disease and giving advice and instruction, under the cardiologist's supervision, on activity and other aspects pertaining to recovery.

A *Clinical Pharmacologist* is very helpful in patient management. Medications are reviewed for correct indications, dosage and usage. Special educational efforts are undertaken with the patient covering the whys and hows of drug usage, including potential side-effects and adverse reactions.

The help of a *Clinical Psychologist* is often critical in changing self-destructive behavior patterns of cigarette smoking, Type A hostile responses, and negative responses to the perceived change in lifestyle as a consequence of development of heart disease. Frequently, for instance, males who have suffered a myocardial infarction have an easily provoked hostility to nurses, doctors and other health care professionals. This seems to be a reaction against their perceived loss of control over their life and now being told all the "dos" and "don'ts" of cardiac rehabilitation. Often, too, the patient may respond to these changes with profound depression and withdrawal. These psychological responses must be recognized and discussed with the patient.

A *Dietician or Nutritionist* is also very helpful throughout all stages of the patients' recovery. With many of the patients requiring cholesterol-restricted diet for coronary risk, salt-restricted for hypertension management, calorie-restricted for diabetes mellitus management, it often takes very innovative dietary management to come up with meals which are palatable and interesting for the patients. Also, a patient may be from an ethnic or socioeconomic background with unusual dietary needs. The dietician must, therefore, have considerable knowledge of ethnic foods and be able to make substitutes which are acceptable to the patient and his spouse.

REFERENCES

1. Price VA: Type A Behavior Pattern. In: *A Model for Research and Practice.* New York: Academic Press, 1982.

2. Kannel WB, Sorlie P, McNamara PM: Prognosis after initial myocardial infarction: The Framingham Study. *Am J Card, 44:*53, 1979.

3. Wenger NK, Hellerstein HK: *Rehabilitation of the Coronary Patient,* Second Edition. New York: John Wiley & Sons, pp. 235-284.

Chapter 14

PROMISES TO KEEP

The past 10 years have seen tremendous strides taken by investigators and clinicians in the diagnosis, treatment and cure of cardiovascular disease. Review of a few of the advancements will serve to illustrate.

We have seen virtual abolition of rheumatic fever by the widespread employment of antibiotics in the treatment of streptococcal infections. Consequently rheumatic valvular heart disease is becoming a rarity in most western industrialized societies.

Pharmacologic therapy can now be employed to manage virtually all degrees of systemic hypertension. Certainly there is continued need for new and better drugs with fewer side-effects, but in the overwhelming majority of patients, a safe, effective, and tolerable drug combination can be found.

Great advances have been made in the diagnosis and management of the manifestations of coronary artery disease. In diagnosis, the advance of safe coronary arteriography must hold the highest rank. In treatment, rapid application of developing knowledge in the use of the three major types of anti-anginal agents has markedly improved the lifestyle of a multitude of angina patients. Coronary bypass grafting, a physiologically sound operation, has provided its own major contribution to relieving the suffering of many patients, as well as, undoubtedly, prolonging the lives of patients with certain types of severe coronary blockage. To one who timorously learned coronary arteriography at a time when one was taught to tippy-toe around these life-giving-and-taking vessels, percutaneous transluminal angioplasty, a very recent member of the cast, appears to be remarkably successful in skilled hands and, because of sprinting technology, appears to have rapidly achieved a high safe plateau.

In recent years, the incidence of the various manifestations of coronary heart disease has appeared to decline. The reason, or reasons, for this are not entirely known. It is possible that some of the above advances have contributed to the decline, but this is difficult to prove. In all probability, the tireless efforts of American Heart Association volunteers in spreading the gospel of risk-factor intervention, and the accelerating national interest in physical fitness have also contributed their share in this hopeful trend.

In the valvular diseases, the technological advances of echocardiography and echo-Doppler have added breathtaking insights into the pathophysiology, diagnosis, and management.

Of course, advances in cardiovascular surgery has leaped and bounded over several previously lethal congenital heart and valvular heart conditions.

For the future, it seems that the major challenges for cardiovascular researchers will be to define more clearly the subcellular mechanisms responsible for heart failure and lethal cardiac arrhythmias and to come up with some pharmacologic, mechanical or ionic means of augmenting this myocardium. At present, in the patient with end-stage heart failure, the only hope, though remote for most, lies in cardiac transplantation. This solution to what is a huge problem is not really a solution, requiring the death of one for the possible survival of another. Also, transplantation is so expensive that it is extremely unlikely that any society will be able to fund a fully comprehensive program without entering the financial realm currently inhabited only by national defense. (Not an illogical hope, but unlikely to ever come to pass.)

Therefore, this author challenges the health professional to set to work on the next great advances in the field of cardiovascular disease, that of solving the riddles of heart failure and lethal cardiac arrhythmias from whatever cause. Once this challenge is met, death from cardiovascular disease will finally take a precipitous drop in the ratings, leaving more room finally for other disease systems to share the inviable position on top of the mortality chart. Perhaps then, medical science can look forward to pushing the life expectancy over the century mark before the end of the 20th century.

INDEX